You

Miracle
Brain

ALSO BY JEAN CARPER

Your Miracle Brain

Maximize Your Brainpower
Boost Your Memory
Lift Your Mood
Improve Your IQ and Creativity
Prevent and Reverse Mental Aging

Jean Carper

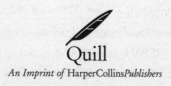

Quill

An Imprint of HarperCollins*Publishers*

A hardcover edition of this book was published in 2000 by HarperCollins Publishers.

YOUR MIRACLE BRAIN. Copyright © 2000 by Jean Carper. All rights reserved. Printed in the United States of America. No part of this book may be used or reproduced in any manner whatsoever without written permission except in the case of brief quotations embodied in critical articles and reviews. For information address HarperCollins Publishers Inc., 10 East 53rd Street, New York, NY 10022.

HarperCollins books may be purchased for educational, business, or sales promotional use. For information please write: Special Markets Department, HarperCollins Publishers Inc., 10 East 53rd Street, New York, NY 10022.

First Quill edition published 2001.

Library of Congress Cataloging-in-Publication Data is available.

ISBN 0-06-098440-6 (pbk.)

03 04 05 ❖/RRD 10 9 8 7 6 5 4

CONTENTS

CONTENTS

CONTENTS

CONTENTS

Part III: Brain Supplements: What to Take for a Miracle Brain

Part IV: How to Keep Vascular Villains from Destroying Your Brain

Postscript: Getting the Miracle Brain You Deserve—Ten Top Strategies

ACKNOWLEDGMENTS

In writing this book, I have been privileged to be able to call upon the best scientific minds of our day in the area of brain research and nutrition. These scientists are exceptional in their ability and willingness to help me interpret the many scientific studies on the subject of the brain, diet, and supplements, so that I can accurately translate the information into what I hope are easily understandable ideas and advice for readers. I want to especially thank several prominent researchers who were the main sources of my fundamental understanding of how nutrition influences the brain. Of course, in the end, the responsibility for the final conclusions and details are mine alone, not theirs.

William Lands, Ph.D., formerly a professor of biochemistry at the University of Illinois at Chicago and now a researcher at the National Institute of Alcohol and Drug Abuse. With my single course in high school chemistry, I would understand a smidgen of what I read about omega–3 fish oils and other fatty acids, if I hadn't had a consummate teacher in Bill Lands to explain it to me in his patient and ever-encouraging manner. I thank him immensely for being my friend and my mentor in the biochemistry of fatty acids for more than a decade.

Jerry Cott, Ph.D., and Joseph Hibbeln, M.D., who hold prominent research positions at the National Institute of

Mental Health. They were always available to provide the latest research information and explanations of brain mechanisms, regarding nutrients and supplements. Their knowledge and their skill at sharing it were simply invaluable.

Denham Harman, M.D., professor emeritus of medicine at the University of Nebraska Medical School. My professional life changed considerably after meeting Denham in 1994, who is the acknowledged father of the free radical theory of aging. He has spent countless hours educating me about free radicals and antioxidants.

Lester Packer, Ph.D., professor of molecular biology at the University of California at Berkeley, and world authority on free radicals and antioxidants. He is a legend for his energy, his encyclopedic scientific knowledge, and his prodigious research. I am very happy to count him among my inner circle of sources of information for this book.

Norman Rosenthal, M.D., a research psychiatrist at the National Institute for Mental Health and the author of books on depression. I first met Norm in 1981 when I was the senior medical correspondent for CNN in Washington, D.C. His invaluable expertise, enthusiasm, and suggestions helped shape this book.

Also, I am grateful for extensive help and information from Andreas Papas, Ph.D., an authority on vitamin E; British psychologist Dr. David Benton; psychologist-researcher Donald Gold; brain and lipids authority Carol Greenwood, Ph.D.; leading vitamin researcher Adrianne Bendich, Ph.D.; and the entire research team at the United States Department of Agriculture Human Nutrition Research Center on Aging at Tufts University, particularly James Joseph, Ph.D., and Ronald Prior, Ph.D. Thanks to Judy McBride, U.S. Department of Agriculture, are also long overdue for her quick responses to requests for information.

I could not have written this book without my researcher, Julie Simons, who kept a steady flow of scientific journal articles coming to me for many months.

And a special thanks to my attorney-agent, Robert Barnett, who cuts through legalese like no one I have ever seen; my editor and associate publisher at HarperCollins, Gladys Justin Carr; and my long-time publicist Edna Farley.

As always—and one more time—I repeat my gratitude to my long-time friend and incomparable editor and television producer, Thea Flaum, for her insightful reading of the manuscript and her endless enthusiasm and encouragement.

INTRODUCTION

Nutritional Neuroscience— the New Frontier

Since the 1960s, researchers have bombarded us with information on everything we can do to keep our heart strong and our arteries clear—what to eat to lower our cholesterol, keep our arteries from clogging, and the rhythms of our heartbeat regular. But what about the brain? It, too, scientists now know, is greatly influenced by what we eat. In fact, few people realize that brain cells are even more sensitive than other body cells to nutrients and dietary chemicals which determine at any moment how your brain functions or malfunctions.

Unquestionably, the brain is our most precious physical possession, the seat of our entire being—our intelligence, personality, our humanity, our mind, and soul. Nothing is more central to a successful and fulfilling life than an optimally functioning brain. Failure to achieve a brain's full intellectual, creative, and emotional potential is a personal tragedy for millions of people, handicapping them from birth to death. Losing one's mind, from psychiatric diseases, nutritional ignorance, and premature aging, is the worst blow to our dignity as human beings. Yet, the brain has received phenomenally little nutritional attention or intervention. For years the brain has been "the forgotten organ," says psychiatrist Turan Itil, clinical professor of medicine at New York University.

Only now is solid scientific advice on what individuals can do to optimize, save, and restore this all-important organ emerging from the world's most highly respected medical and research institutions.

Medical journals are exploding with the news, heralding a new age of the brain. As the brain firmly replaces brawn in the twenty-first century information society, interest in how to scientifically boost brain functioning is surging. With the dawning of the realization that the brain is our primary resource and that intelligence is the currency of our present and future, more people worry whether their brains will measure up. As *Newsweek* commented recently in an article titled "Brain Boosters" (reporting a new study on the success of ginkgo in treating Alzheimer's disease): "Life in the Information Age strains everyone's processing capacity—and countless Americans are turning to supplements to improve, or at least preserve, whatever they've got."

Also, the aging of the population is spurring a new realization that a vital body without a vital brain is meaningless. By the year 2030 we will have eighty million Americans over age 65. The number of us with memory and brain problems threatens to become a public health nightmare unless we take action, say experts. "We must start paying as much or more attention to the brain as we do to the heart," says Dr. Itil. He favors establishment of "memory centers" (like heart centers) to test for brain function and memory decline after middle age and administer appropriate nutrients and memory enhancers to prevent further brain deterioration and degeneration.

At long last, the brain is becoming the new focus of cutting-edge nutritional research worldwide, as scientists search for and discover fascinating ways to alter brain chemistry with supplements, diet, and other lifestyle changes. Their discoveries reveal how to keep the brain functioning at peak power for an entire lifetime—from boosting the capacities of fetal brains to preventing and reversing brain breakdown as we grow older. This new emphasis on enhancing and saving the brain has even spurred a new medical speciality called "nutritional neuroscience" with a new scientific journal of the same name.

A recent article in *Psychology Today* summed it up: "The idea that the right foods, or the natural neurochemicals they contain, can enhance mental capabilities—help you concentrate, tune sensorimotor skills, keep you motivated, magnify memory, speed reaction times, defuse stress, perhaps even prevent brain aging—is not idle speculation. Nutritional neuroscience, as it's called, is barely in its infancy, but it's already turning up some head-turning findings."

This fast-moving ultra-fascinating research on how you can influence your own brain functioning has encouraged me to explore the latest scientific evidence, revealing how everyone can use nutrients, vitamins, supplements, and other lifestyle factors to increase brain power, achieve and maintain a happy state of mind, and prevent or reverse brain deterioration related to aging or neurological diseases. This extends to what a pregnant woman can eat to ensure that her future child will have a high IQ and what an older person can take to bring back failing memory, as well as what people can do at all ages in between to enjoy optimal brain functioning. The result is *Your Miracle Brain*.

This book looks at the latest research on some of the oldest brain-modifiers, such as caffeine and sugar, as well as some of the newest synthetic memory boosters, such as phosphatidylserine (PS) and ginkgo. It reexamines the power of common vitamins in regulating mood and cognitive functioning in light of the latest research. Essentially, *Your Miracle Brain*, based on a new knowledge of the brain's plasticity, is a cutting-edge guide to everything you can do to enhance brain power at all ages, making you smarter and more creative, as well as to prevent the loss of brain power as you grow older. It is never too early or too late to improve the physiology of your brain, boosting its functioning to its optimal intellectual and emotional heights. This book tells you how and why you should start now.

For the first time, science suggests ways you can actually improve the biological structure and electrochemical wiring of your brain to help you realize your optimal potential for happiness, achievement, and fulfillment.

PART 1

WELCOME TO THE AGE OF THE MIRACLE BRAIN

POPULAR MYTH: You are born with a genetically determined brain of a certain size and potential, and that's it. There's little or no way to alter its capabilities and functioning; thus, your chances in life are predestined, your fate sealed.

NEW SCIENTIFIC REALITY: The brain is a growing, changing organ, its capabilities and vitality dependent to a large degree on how you nourish and treat it. Thus, you can dramatically influence your brain's functioning and your own destiny. The long-neglected brain is now being exposed to intense biological scrutiny, and the news is good for all of us.

Good-bye, "Brain as Machine"
In every century, philosophers, scientists, clergy, and scholars put their particular spin on the nature of the brain. In the mid 1700s, a British philosopher described the brain

as "an ingenious system of vibrating hollow tubes," similar to a church organ. In the industrial age, the appropriate metaphor is brain as machine, currently that ultimate information processor, the computer—hardwired, forged of immutable metal and chips to be programmed, with a preordained memory and capacity.

But new brain discoveries render the metaphor unsuitable. If the demands on your computer outstrip its capabilities, it becomes junk. It does not grow a few more chips, nor rev up its inner byte resources to improve memory or performance. No, its physical structure is decreed forever by circumstances of its birth in some computer factory. You can kick it, pour nutrients over it, make it listen to music, give it smart drugs, but it does not get smarter. Not so with a real, living brain.

The notion of brain as computer or machine is a relic of yesterday's science. Exciting new investigations of the brain show it to be a growing, ever-changing massive complexity of cells, a miraculous living organ malleable by external and internal influences. Just as the structure and function of the heart changes—improving or deteriorating—in response to diet, drugs, and exercise, so do those of the brain.

Neuroscientists now know the brain is an organ of mind-boggling plasticity—like the rest of your body, dynamic, not "fixed" for life. Larry Squire, professor of neuroscience at the University of California at San Diego and past president of the national Society for Neuroscience, has said: "If you could use a video camera to watch the brain respond to experiences, I have no doubt you would see it growing, retracting, reshaping."

"The most important thing is to realize that the brain is growing and changing all the time," agrees leading brain researcher Bruce McEwen at New York's Rockefeller University.

"The chemical composition of the neurons themselves is changing, and hence there is no separate and unchanging hardware, in contrast to a programmable range of software." —Susan Greenfield, *The Human Brain: A Guided Tour*, 1997

Until recently, we have known little about the biological architecture of the brain compared with other organs, such as the liver, kidney, and heart. Why? Very simple, says British neurologist Richard S.J. Frackowiak at London's Institute of Neurology, in a fascinating article in *Daedalus*, published in 1998 by the American Academy of Arts and Sciences. The brain was simply not available for examination. Hidden in "a relatively impenetrable box, the skull," the human brain could not be readily probed or excised during life, but only after death. All knowledge about how the brain functioned was remote, deduced from human behavior. That began to change in 1972 with the arrival of computerized tomography (CT) scans and later positron-emission tomography (PET) scans which could turn out clear images of brain anatomy and metabolism and track chemicals as they made their way through elaborate pathways in the brain. With this remarkable new noninvasive technology, our interest definitely perked up. For the first time, we humans can now begin to understand in remarkable detail the structure and function of the source of our unique place in the universe—how our brain works and how we can make it work even better. The ancient mystery is yielding to twenty-first century knowledge.

Fantastic Pictures of the Living Brain

At one time, the only way scientists could study the anatomy of the brain was by examining dead brain tissue. Of course, they still study autopsied brain slices under electron microscopes. But the study of dead brain cells has given way to exquisite observations of live brain cells in action. Much of the revolutionary thinking about the brain is made possible by new technology that allows scientists to peer inside the brain as it is thinking, processing information, learning new things, consolidating memory and expressing anger, depression, even having hallucinations and psychotic episodes. The remarkable new field of brain imaging can reveal even the voices of demons lurking in the brains of schizophrenics. For example, the October 1995 issue of *Time* magazine showed a "snapshot of a hallucination," a freeze-frame of a brain with six red-orange blobs, indicating hot spots of intense activity captured on a PET scan. The hot colors occurred every time a twenty-three-year-old paranoid schizophrenic pressed a button to signal he was having a hallucination of disembodied heads shouting abuse and commands at him. These brain images not only confirm brain activity and help diagnose mental problems, but also offer concrete evidence of beneficial brain changes induced by various nutrients, drugs, hormones, and herbal treatments.

Sophisticated colorful 3-D brain images can trace the routes of neurotransmitters as they congregate to elicit mood changes and lay down long-term memory. Scientists using brain images can witness the amount of blood flow to areas of the brain and how much energy the brain uses—how it burns glucose—to perform a task. Generally, the greater the blood flow and the more glucose consumed, the harder the brain is working. In some studies, scientists observe that an older brain must work harder than a younger brain to process or retrieve the same information. Also, brain images show that the brains of adults and children with attention deficit disorder have abnormalities in the way they burn glucose. Similarly, images show that schizophrenic brains are different from normal brains.

Using imaging, scientists can see the neurotransmitter dopamine rise in the brains of men playing video games; they can record centers of activation in the brains of cocaine users, thus pinpointing addiction hot spots. They can chart intense activity in the limbic system of the brain during a panic attack. They can view flashes of red and yellow in the brain when you simply imagine numbers in your mind. They can map brain activity in response to music—whether you hear a pleasing melody or discordant notes. They have even located the brain center of perfect pitch. They can document the changing fatty composition of brain cell membranes and measure both the destruction and the proliferation of new brain cells.

> **BOTTOM LINE:** *Much dogma is being thrown on the trash heap after being scrutinized by new techniques of sophisticated brain imaging, including functional MRI (magnetic resonance imaging), PET (positron-emission tomography) and the most recent, SPECT (single photon emission-computed tomography), that can track the workings of a living human brain. This has ushered in a new era of the "biology of the brain."*

Welcome to the world of the miracle brain!

Enter the New Biology of the Brain

Little by little, just in the last decade, the concept of a "fixed forever" brain has been abandoned. And discoveries are happening at a whirlwind pace. Pioneering research has proved the ever-changing nature of the brain: Brain cells continually produce new dendrites and receptors, grow

THE AMAZING NERVE CELL

At the center of our memory, our intellect, our emotions, our identity are nerve cells called neurons. A neuron is a unique creation with a small, roundish body and nucleus with offshoots of a complex bushy network of sinewy branches or dendrites and a single long nerve fiber or axon. The dendrites are studded with countless surface "receptors" that receive incoming signals from other neurons. The signals streak down the dendritic branches to the cell body where the information is processed and then passed on to the axon for transmission to other neurons through their dendritic connections. At the end of the tip end of the axon is a storage "terminal" with tiny sacs full of chemicals called neurotransmitters. As neurotransmitters are released, messages flash across junctions or "synapses" at the end of the axon of one cell to specific receptors on another. These synapses are the message transmission centers of the neurons' business— the way cells talk to each other.

Each neuron can have myriad synapses and thus communicate with hundreds of thousands of other neurons in microseconds. It's logical that the more and better connections or synapses and dendrites a nerve cell has, the greater its capacity for transmitting messages and processing information, which translates into heightened intelligence and better mental functioning. The astonishing news: You can create more connections—synapses, dendrites and receptors— through diet, supplements, and mental and physical activity.

new synapses, or communication junctions, and alter the essence of the neurotransmitter soup that stimulates brain activity. And even adult brains can grow brand new cells!

Most exciting of all, researchers are now answering the big question: How can you influence this vast potential that looms inside your head? For the first time in human history, scientists are beginning to understand how profoundly a person can influence the factors that control brain functioning—through food, supplements, and simple lifestyle changes, including mental and physical exercise.

At one time, for example, it was thought that the brain and central nervous system were not readily affected by diet. The mistaken assumption: that the blood brain barrier was designed to discriminate carefully among nutrients in the blood so as not to continually upset the balance or homeostasis of the central nervous system. New research shows that nutrients, including glucose and fat, can have an almost immediate impact on brain cells and brain functioning, producing rapid changes in mood and monumental changes in long-term behavior. For years vitamins, for example, were regarded as merely "cofactors" needed for enzymatic reactions, notes Professor Chandan Prasad of Louisiana State University Medical Center and editor-in-chief of the journal *Nutritional Neuroscience*. Now vitamins are hailed as potent antioxidants with enormous impact on all cells, including those of the brain, he says. Pursuing the mysteries of how the brain depends on food to supply chemicals to synthesize and regulate neurotransmitters, sending messages zipping through the brain, is frontier research. It's almost mind-boggling to realize that the emergence from the dark ages of blind ignorance of the connection between brain functioning, behavior, and diet is but thirty years old—a mere eye-blink in the world of science.

Brain Fact: The number of synaptic connections in the brain has been roughly estimated at 100,000,-000,000,000 (a hundred billion).

The Neurotransmitter Revolution

Some of the most thrilling discoveries about how the brain works, and how you can influence thought and behavior with food and supplements, come from new knowledge about the activity of neurotransmitter systems. It is these brain chemicals (so far about fifty have been identified) that substantially define who you are at every microsecond of your life. Flashing through neurons one by one, neurotransmitters lay down biochemical highways that carry your every thought and feeling through the brain's vast neuronal network. Without neurotransmitters, the lights in the brain would go out; they are the biochemical electrification system of your brain. They are the essence of your memory, intelligence, creativity, and mood.

Until recently, the idea that food might profoundly and rapidly influence brain chemistry was considered scientifically ludicrous. Scientists thought the brain, of all organs, was particularly protected from the random permutations of nutrient invasions. It turns out the brain is uniquely responsive to food chemicals.

> *"The ability of a meal's composition to affect the production of brain chemicals distinguishes the brain from all other organs. The crucial compounds that regulate other organs are largely independent of whatever was in the last meal we ate—but not the brain."*
> —Richard Wurtman, research-psychiatrist, MIT

In the late 1970s, a team of researchers at the Massachusetts Institute of Technology, led by Dr. Richard Wurtman, had the first glimmering that food constituents could mimic drugs in regulating neurotransmitters, causing changes in brain activity and behavior. Since then research into the nutritional origins and workings of neurotransmitters and their potential impact on personality and behavior has led to revolutionary findings.

The radical conclusion: The type of neurotransmitters your neurons make and release and their ultimate destiny within the brain depend greatly on what you eat. Obviously, that makes food a very big regulator of the brain.

The thinking goes this way: Your brain cells require certain nutrients as building blocks to make various neurotransmitters. Thus, the availability of a specific nutrient can dictate the levels and potency of a particular neurotransmitter. For example, brain cells need tryptophan, an amino acid in foods, to readily create serotonin, the good-mood messenger. Similarly, choline, concentrated in egg yolk, is required to make the neurotransmitter acetylcholine, critical for memory. The brain makes the neurotransmitter dopamine, essential for proper motor coordination, from an amino acid, tyrosine, found in high- protein containing foods. Other nutrients such as folic acid and fish oil can help determine the amount, character, and functioning of brain-altering neurotransmitters. When brain cells don't get enough of the right nutrients, neurotransmitter systems can go awry with disastrous consequences.

One way memory is destroyed, as in dementia and Alzheimer's, is through a disruption of the neurotransmitter systems. Initially, researchers held neurons responsible for not synthesizing and releasing enough neurotransmitters. The solution: Devise ways to flood brain cells with more neurotransmitters, which is the rationale behind many drug treatments for dementia and mood disorders. But scientists now know it's more complex than neuro-

SEROTONIN: ONE MIGHTY MESSENGER

The most extensively studied neurotransmitter is serotonin. It influences practically every aspect of brain life, helping shape your mood, energy level, memory, outlook on life. Antidepressants, such as Prozac, work by enhancing serotonin in the brain. People with low levels of serotonin are more vulnerable to depression, impulsive acts, alcoholism, suicide, aggression, and violence. Scientists can even make lab animals more aggressive by altering their brain serotonin levels.

Interestingly, women synthesize brain serotonin at half the rate of men, which may help explain why women are more prone to depression. Serotonin circuits also grow weaker with age because neurons lose receptors needed to activate serotonin. According to one study, the brains of sixty-five-year olds had 60 percent fewer serotonin receptors of a specific type than the brains of thirty-year-olds. Thus, the effect of serotonin lessens with age, increasing the tendency to depression.

Additionally, serotonin can heighten memory and help protect brain cells from a process called "excito-toxicity" that destroys neurons. Thus, ample serotonin actually helps prevent brain damage as you age! Many supplements, vitamins, nutrients, and fatty acids help enhance and regulate serotonin activity.

"A person's mood is like a symphony, and serotonin is like the conductor's baton." —James Stockard, psychiatrist, Northwestern University

transmitter shortage. New research focuses on the receiving apparatus of nerve cells—how plentiful and "sensitive" dendritic receptors are at capturing and processing neurotransmitters. No matter how much of a neurotransmitter roams the brain, if receptors are not "activated" to pass the message on, it stops dead. Abnormalities in receptors can cause widespread trouble. In the brains of Alzheimer's patients, for example, the number of receptors for acetylcholine declines as does the receptors' ability to transmit messages. One new research direction: how to create more receptors and manipulate their sensitivity.

The important point is this: The composition of these neurotransmitters and the functional biochemistry of the receptors are changing all the time—and some of that change is dependent on what you eat and what you do.

Until very recently, we have been imprisoned by a scientifically fallacious view of the brain, proclaiming it beyond our control. The rapid eradication of that concept in the last few years is astonishing. After thirty-five years of pioneering research on the nature of the brain, Marian Diamond, Ph.D., of the University of California at Berkeley, can now say with breathtaking authority: "The brain can decide its own destiny." The revolutionary new knowledge about the brain is so recent—occurring only in the last six or seven years—that most people don't even realize the old misconceptions are dead and buried, says leading brain researcher Marilyn Albert of the Harvard Medical School.

Basically, two pivotal notions about the nature of the brain have been nullified. One is that the brain ceases to grow and change after childhood. The second is that the brain steadily loses brain cells after age twenty or so and consequently relentlessly declines in mental capacities.

No one questioned that young brains grew, changed, and

developed. But scientists thought older brains lost the capacity to grow, and were fixed and static after puberty. It's now known that brain cells can sprout new dendrites and new synapses, forming new communication networks, at any age! Thus, although everyone is born with a fixed number of brain cells, that innate figure does not define mental capacity; what counts is the proliferation of connections throughout life. Brains with fewer cells can have just as much, or more, mental capacity than larger brains, depending on the lushness of neurons. The idea that a massive and progressive loss of neurons is an inevitable consequence of aging has also been thoroughly disproved.

"The process by which the brain is 'wired' and even 'rewired' is referred to as plasticity. This means that the brain is always changing and repairing itself. . . . We now know that even the brains of adults are constantly changing and being rewired." —Russell L. Blaylock, M.D., University of Mississippi Medical Center

Old Brains Don't Die: They Just Lose Power

Until very recently, the prevailing dogma was that neurons died off by the thousands, even millions, every day throughout the brain in the normal course of adult life, and that the older a person, the faster the cells disappeared. Neuroscientists believed that by old age, as much as 40 percent of the brain's cells could be destroyed by normal aging. Such wholesale loss, it was thought, could only result in a brain with diminished capacity. In other words, we all were doomed to failing memory and fading intellectual capacity; "senility" was a real possibility for virtually everyone who lived long enough.

But new, more sophisticated examinations of healthy,

normal brains show how wrong that idea was. Indeed, although some cells in certain parts of the brain disappear with aging, it is far from a devastating blow. In fact, the loss of neurons in the areas of the brain where it matters most—the cortex, the seat of memory and thinking—is minimal in aging brains undamaged by disease, says Harvard's Dr. Albert. Loss of neurons with age is more apt to occur deep in the brain where damage is relatively small, chemical in nature, less significant and more amenable to fixing.

"We used to think that you lost brain cells every day of your life everywhere in the brain. That's just not so— you do have some loss with healthy aging, but not so dramatic, and in very selective brain areas."
—Marilyn Albert, brain researcher, Harvard Medical School

"It's a colossal myth that people lose millions of brain cells every day as they age." —Thomas H. McNeil, University of Southern California

More commonly, new research shows, the aging brain seems to experience a power shortage, a fading of function, not a complete loss. "What we think happens is the signaling properties [the transmission of messages] change in aging," says James Joseph, Tufts University neuroscientist. "Instead of saying you lose cells so there are fewer messages, we now say: There's probably the same number of messages, they just can't get through."

In other words, the circuitry of cells functions less efficiently. Tiny hitches in cellular communication, magnified billions of times, can add up to discernible mental deficits, such as failing memory, inability to learn rapidly, faulty motor coordination. Under the old theory, the building is crumbling and weakening; under the new one, the wiring and pipes within the building are less functional and efficient.

In human terms, it is far more optimistic to address and correct the latter than the former. A brain that has severely shrunk may need massive restructuring. A brain whose machinery is simply not working well may need mere tinkering. A collapsing, disintegrating brain leaves little hope for significant salvation; a brain with wiring problems that erode the integrity of the brain's circuitry may be fixed to the degree that the internal communication functions can be restored. In short, as you age, you need to find ways to boost the efficiency of brain cell functioning, instead of worrying about lost neurons, and to avoid diseases that can damage your brain.

It now seems clear that the amount of brain mass is not a true test of a brain's quality. Scientists used to think so, but now they believe how elaborate the neuronal networks are and the strength of their connections and circuitry really count more than the brute number of brain cells. In short, how well a brain conducts electrochemical business between cells appears more crucial to memory, intelligence, and mood than the total number of neurons tucked under the skull. This is good news, because old brains appear just as adept as young brains at growing new brain cell connections, suggest results of animal experiments by Dr. Carl Cotman at the University of California at Irvine. Researchers even find evidence of new brain cell connections in individuals in the early stages of Alzheimer's.

BOTTOM LINE: *What really matters as you age is not the size of your brain or how many neurons are left, but how it is wired, and what you can do to preserve or rejuvenate the wiring if necessary.*

In the last few years scientists have junked their old beliefs and come up with a revisionist view of the aging brain. "Most notions about aging and the brain are based on folklore rather than fact," said Dr. Zaven Khachaturian, former director of research at the National Institute on Aging, as quoted in *The New York Times*. "If you really study aging carefully and look at it in the absence of disease, there is no reason to believe that aging per se leads to decline and loss of cognitive and intellectual activities."

Still, the undeniable reality is that normal brains as they age do shrink ever so slightly; the speed of processing new information and retrieving stored information slows down and short term memory is less sharp. Such changes may be disconcerting, but they are usually not an indication of progressive mental decline or Alzheimer's disease.

So Your Brain Shrinks, So What?

Dr. Stanley Rapoport, at the National Institute on Aging, has used PET scans to study the brains of people ages twenty to ninety-three. Fortunately, brain scans decidedly show that a healthy brain does *not* suffer a massive wipe-out of neurons, he says. Between ages twenty and seventy, the average loss of brain mass is about 10 percent, a mere two-tenths of a percent a year. Relinquishing even a smidgen of your brain to aging may seem alarming. But in reality, Dr. Rapoport says, it may signify little in diminished mental performance. Most importantly, it does not mean a significant downturn in intellectual function or that Alzheimer's is in your future.

The anatomical and metabolic changes, Dr. Rapoport notes, that occur in normal aging brains are "very subtle," and may cause only slight diminution in mental activity. He finds that the loss often occurs in brain regions not critical for intellectual functioning. Moreover, older brains have wondrous ways of compensating, for example, by expanding synaptic elements to close the gap when synapses are lost, reorganizing to recruit other neuronal regions, and simply working harder.

What normal aging people typically perceive as failing memory—"it's on the tip of my tongue" syndrome—is not a blow-out, but a slow-down. The most common age-related brain glitch seems to be in the speed of processing information. Research by Dr. Rapoport and others find that older brains do react more slowly and take more time to store, recall, and process information. Retrieval of information slows down about 10 percent after age seventy.

Older individuals, no matter how intelligent or how intact their general memory, cannot match younger people in mental tests involving processing unfamiliar information. Even acknowledged aged geniuses, still at the top of their form as symphony conductors, for example, score lower than the least mentally adroit college students on certain tests of matching digits with symbols, and other spatial or arithmetical tasks. But accuracy of memory and verbal fluency need not be diminished by age.

Given time, healthy old brains can usually retrieve information just as well, albeit not as quickly, as young brains. "They get it right, but it just takes longer," says Dr. Rapoport.

Besides a slowdown in mental processing, the most noticeable casualty of normal aging seems to be short-term memory—the ability to recall newly learned information, such as phone numbers and names—say experts. But James McGaugh, director of the Center for the Neurobiology of Learning and Memory at the University of California at Irvine, compares such loss to farsightedness, a nondebilitating natural part of aging.

Further, in one type of mental activity, age brings an advantage. It's called "crystallized" intelligence—the accumulation of specialized knowledge over the years that comes from life experiences and requires a large memory bank, well-honed verbal abilities, and judgment. This is very different from so-called "fluid" intelligence that blesses the young and demands speed at dealing with novel learning situations. Whereas old brains cannot keep up with young ones in "fluid" intelligence, they excel in the mental realm of "crystallized" knowledge or intelligence.

Old Brains Don't Shrink Faster

You need not fear that the rate of brain shrinkage will pick up as you get older if you remain in good health, says neurologist Jeffrey Kaye, M.D., director of the Aging and Alzheimer's Center at Oregon Health Sciences University. Your brain at age eighty-five should be just as voluminous as it is at age sixty-five, he says. He used MRI scans to measure brain volume in forty-five healthy individuals over a period of five years. The *rate* of brain shrinkage did not accelerate after age sixty-five. Surprisingly, Dr. Kaye even found that the volume of some cortical regions of the brain *increased* during old age! This supports the idea that new neurons can spring up, even in old brains. "This study suggests we can age normally forever," he says.

In earlier days, Dr. Kaye says, researchers thought brains shrank the older you got because they mistakenly measured the size of diseased Alzheimer's brains, which were shrinking, thinking them normal. Current imaging techniques enable investigators to spot Alzheimer's much earlier and eliminate the inclusion of these diseased brains in such research.

Thus, it is a subtle slowdown in the electrochemical

MEN'S BRAINS SHRINK FASTER

For unknown reasons, male brains undergo more changes with aging than women's. Indeed, in a brain-imaging study of 330 healthy people ages sixty-five to ninety-five, Dr. Edward Coffey, chairman of the psychiatry department at the Henry Ford Health System in Detroit, found that men's brains shrink faster with age than women's brains. One possible reason: Estrogen may protect women's brains. Dr. Coffey also said this doesn't mean men show increased cognitive decline, because brain shrinkage does not necessarily mean significantly lower intellectual functioning.

communication network rather than the massive death of brain cells that seems to account for the typical measurable decline in mental processing that comes with age.

PET scans do show that the rate of blood flow in the gray matter of the front cortex starts to lessen around age fifty, and that older brains must usually work harder in burning glucose to process information. There is a reduction in the efficiency of energy production in the mitochondria of brain cells with age. Some shrinkage and mental problems are also due to vascular problems, including high blood pressure and reduced blood flow. High blood pressure reduces the size of brain and can cause subtle injuries to brain tissue, resulting in cognitive decline.

The primary reason memory and intellectual abilities seem to fade in older people is due far more to disease than to normal aging, experts now believe. "The distinction between disease and aging has not been made clear enough," says Dr. Peter Davies, director of the Alzheimer's brain bank at the Albert Einstein College of Medicine in New York. Alzheimer's is not a natural condition to be feared by everyone, he has said. If you can keep your brain free of disease, it can function perfectly well for a long lifetime.

Indeed, a major new study of the cognitive status of older people by researchers at the Center for Aging and Health at the University of California, Davis, found that mental decline resulted from disease—including diabetes, thickened carotid arteries, high systolic blood pressure, and early Alzheimer's—and not from simply being old. "Cognitive decline is not a normal part of aging for the majority of elderly people," declares Mary N. Haan, director of the center. Fully 70 percent of 5888 people over age sixty-five suffered no decline in memory or other mental faculties, as shown by standard tests, over a seven-year period, she says. Significant loss of cognitive function happened *only* in those with serious atherosclerosis or diabetes and/or a specific gene for dementia and Alzheimer's. Those with both disease and the gene were eight times more apt to show signs of intellectual decline than those without disease or the gene.

Prime Enemy: Free Radicals

There is a specific hazard to the brain from aging. It is also the primary root cause of disease that damages the brain. It stems from routine chemical reactions that take place in the depths of each cell—primarily in the cell's thousands of energy factories called "mitochondria." Denham Harman, M.D., emeritus professor of medicine at the University of Nebraska and the father of the free radical theory of aging, explains that throughout life all your cells, including your brain cells, are bombarded by attacks from unstable chemicals called oxygen free radicals that are the result of breathing, eating, simply being alive. When the mito-chondria burn oxygen to make energy for cells, byproducts called oxygen free radicals are thrown off. Typically, they are chemically transformed into missiles that attack the walls of the mitochondria and into toxins that penetrate the interior, even the DNA, and membranes of the cells themselves. Over the years free radical damage accumu-lates in cells and their energy production slows down. In nerve cells, attacks by free radicals cause dendrites to retract and synapses to vanish, dramatically cutting back on a cell's communication abilities. Eventually, free radical damage threatens neuronal survival.

The longer you live, the more free radicals your cells generate, making you more susceptible to simple age-related brain damage as well as degenerative brain disor-ders. Such free radical damage may disrupt normal mental function. In vulnerable brains, years of free radical batter-ing may destroy neurons, ending in Alzheimer's disease, Parkinson's, ALS (Lou Gehrig's disease), or another form of degenerative brain disease. The amount of cumulative damage and potential intellectual decline depend greatly on the strength of your antioxidant defenses—or free rad-ical fighters—say many experts.

In Dr. Harman's view, aging itself is a disease of vary-ing severity. Some brains age much faster than others due to excessive free radical damage, much of it needless and preventable, he says. That explains why some brains are more aged and dysfunctional than other brains—why some normal people lose their memory and others don't. The best way to avoid and even reverse these age-induced brain deficits, according to Dr. Harman and many other researchers, is to get more antioxidants into your brain to neutralize the destructive free radicals. Such antioxidants rush to a free radical and, like a science-fiction laser, vaporize it. This strategy has produced thrilling results, identifying antioxidants as one of the most promising ways to save your brain. Boosting antioxidants and antioxidant activity has prevented and *reversed* memory loss in aged animals and even retarded the progression of Alzheimer's in humans! (For more on free radicals and antioxidants, see pages 000).

> *"Aging of the nervous system appears to involve a lifetime of insults, many of which center around a common process: free radical generation and injury."* — Russell L. Blaylock, University of Mississippi Medical Center

Is It Aging or Alzheimer's?

Where does normal brain aging end and Alzheimer's disease take over? Will all of us eventually get Alzheimer's if we live long enough? Despite dramatic advances in the last few years in understanding brain changes involved in Alzheimer's, important aspects of the disease's true nature are still very shadowy. Most experts, however, believe Alzheimer's is a distinct progressive pathological disease, related to aging, but not the end-stage of normal aging. In short, it's not an inevitable consequence of aging. "Clearly people who live to a hundred and a hundred and ten years of age show no evidence of Alzheimer's when we look at their brains," says Dr. Mark Mattson, a leading researcher at the University of Kentucky. "Not everybody will develop Alzheimer's."

According to Dr. Mattson, an aging brain and an Alzheimer's brain have similarities. Indeed, aging is the number one risk factor for Alzheimer's; both aged brains and Alzheimer's brains show signs of free radical damage. But an Alzheimer's brain has distinct patterns of neuronal destruction, not seen in ordinary nondiseased brains

IT'S NEVER TOO EARLY TO
SAVE YOUR BRAIN

When do you have to start worrying about a loss of brain power with age? According to Denham Harman, M.D., emeritus professor of medicine at the University of Nebraska and the father of the free-radical theory of aging, the process sets in even before you are born— in the womb. His early experiments show that pregnant mice given antioxidants had offspring that aged more slowly. Overwhelmingly, research shows that animals fed antioxidants for a lifetime stay healthier as they age; they suffer less chronic disease, have better mental abilities, and live longer. In Dr. Harman's view, the earlier you start to care for your brain, the less it will deteriorate through the years and the better you can expect it to function at all ages.

Alzheimer's doesn't begin when it is diagnosed. Nor does so-called normal age-related memory loss. Loss of brain power, scientists say, begins years earlier and mainly results from gradual undetectable hits on brain cells, hits that go unrepaired and lead to screwups in the brain's circuitry, possibly neuronal death.

Dr. Harman points to a critical age of twenty-eight when antioxidant defenses decline significantly, making you vulnerable to age-related damage. So if you haven't been conscientious in caring for your brain before then, it's definitely time to start.

Paul D. Coleman at the University of Rochester describes the diseased nerve cells from Alzheimer's patients as filled with "black neurofibrillary tangles," material that accumulates in the cell and is "basically choking it to death." Harvard's Dr. Albert notes that Alzheimer's begins in the area of the hippocampus and spreads to other areas of the brain, killing brain cells as it goes and leaving its victim increasingly incapacitated.

Thus, Alzheimer's is far beyond normal aging. Something else happens to trigger the disease. Provocateurs—possibly "genetic alterations," immune dysfunction, metabolic defects, environmental toxins, or other factors—are required to induce the distinctive brain configurations and the steep progressive decline in mental functioning typical of Alzheimer's. Millions of dollars are going into research to identify—and eventually control—the mysterious factors that initiate a brain to Alzheimer's.

About 4 percent of the population between ages sixty-five and seventy-four develop Alzheimer's. The figure jumps to about 50 percent after age eighty-five.

Unquestionably, Alzheimer's brains are different, showing massive loss of cells. Harvard neuroscientist B.T. Hyman and colleagues have measured the number of neurons in the brains of individuals who showed absolutely no signs of intellectual decline at the time of death, and in mentally impaired individuals diagnosed with Alzheimer's disease. The neurons were in the regions of the brain related to memory function and higher-order information processing. The astonishing finding: In the age range from sixty to one hundred, there was "no apparent neuronal loss due to normal aging;" those who were intellectually intact did not show any significant decline in the number of neurons. In contrast, those with Alzheimer's disease had drastic losses of neurons: from a 20 percent decline in those mildly impaired to 70 percent in those severely impaired.

Some Brains Don't Quit

On the other hand, some astonishing new findings show how incredibly resilient the human brain is in the face of danger. It appears, in fact, that brains can endure seemingly monumental damage before becoming dysfunctional. You may seem mentally sound until the day you die, but an autopsy of your brain may show signs of structural damage characteristic of Alzheimer's, according to William R. Markesbery and colleagues at the University of Kentucky's Sanders-Brown Center on Aging. In a new study, Dr. Markesbery discovered that about *half* of a large group of elderly, well-educated persons, who showed no signs of intellectual decline at the time of death, actually had brains with "plaques and tangles" warranting a diagnosis of Alzheimer's! In fact, only 17 percent of the subjects showed no signs of degenerative brain changes. So how can you be cognitively normal and still have a damaged brain? Apparently, say experts, the individuals managed to recruit undamaged brain cells and redundant circuitry in the brain to carry on.

The bottom line: Damage from free radical chemicals is a prime culprit in both ordinary aging deficits in the brain and Alzheimer's. The difference: "Initiating" factors, some genetic, prime vulnerable brains to develop Alzheimer's. Finding those "initiating" factors could relieve the extreme national fear and suffering generated by Alzheimer's. Another top priority: discovering ways to delay the potential devastation of accelerated aging as well as the major degenerative brain diseases—Alzheimer's, Parkinson's, ALS, and Huntington's.

Proof of the Unthinkable: Regeneration

Despite the revolutionary new view of the brain's plasticity, one dogma remained sacred until very recently. The hallowed consensus was that a fully developed adult brain could never grow new cells. A dead brain cell was lost and gone forever, never to be replaced. Thus, the brain could never regenerate itself, fill in the cellular gaps destroyed by Parkinson's, Alzheimer's, alcoholism, strokes, brain injuries, and the aging process. Experts believed any hole in the brain's basic cellular structure was irreparable. The Seventh Age of Shakespeare could never be reversed. There was no Lazarus working inside the brain.

Now, thanks to a group of visionary neuroscientists, that idea, too, has bit the dust, leading to thrilling new prospects of brain regrowth, expansion, recovery, and rejuvenation.

Neuroscientist Fred Gage at the Salk Institute for Biological Studies in La Jolla, California, says as far back as 1965 animal research suggested brains could create new neurons (neurogenesis), but the finding so contradicted mainstream conviction, it was ignored. Gage and colleagues took up the challenge in the early 1990s and found they could grow stem cells from adult rat brains in test tubes. In 1996 they proved new neurons were also being born in the hippocampus of the brains of animals throughout their lives—even into very old age! (The hippocampus is the processing center for much memory and learning, and is usually the major target of damage in Alzheimer's disease.)

Then scientists showed it was happening not only in small animals, but also in the brains of our humanlike cousins, monkeys. In early 1998 Drs. Elizabeth Gould of Princeton University and Bruce S. McEwen of Rockefeller University reported that new brain cells were showing up every day by the thousands in the hippocampus of mature marmoset monkeys. Dr. Gould suspects old brain cells die expressly to make room for new ones. "It mandates new ways of thinking about the brain," she said.

Also astonishing was the finding that when the monkeys were under stress, frightened and gushing out cortisol, their production of new brain cells decreased rapidly and dramatically. Scientists say the same thing is likely in human brains.

The real coup came in a breakthrough study in late 1998 by Dr. Gage and Peter Eriksson at the Sahlgrenska University Hospital in Goteborg, Sweden, demonstrating conclusively that human brains, too, give birth to new brain cells, even in old age. The two investigators identified mature new nerve cells in the deep-brain structure, the hippocampus, in autopsies of five patients, all over age fifty; two were past seventy. Their brain cells in that area were dividing, thus spawning new cells. "It's an exciting discovery, the isolation of a specific part of the human brain where you actually caught a glimpse of new cells being produced," agreed Rockefeller University's McEwen.

This unprecedented discovery gives hope that the brain can spawn new neurons to regenerate itself and repair broken circuitry caused by aging, damage, or disease. "What we're saying," according to Dr. Gage, "is that the same programs that are present during [early development] are persisting throughout life. Things we thought were ending are not ending, they're just continuing at a slower rate."

When Dead Is Not Dead

Further, the idea that neurons die quickly and irreversibly within minutes of being deprived of oxygen and glucose has been challenged. Investigators at the Netherlands Institute for Brain Research in Amsterdam have resuscitated neurons in the brains of humans who have been dead for up to eight hours! They found that presumed-dead neurons from thirty postmortem human brains, when bathed in artificial cerebrospinal fluid, literally came back to life and recovered the ability to burn oxygen and transport nerve signals along axons. Researchers speculate that some unknown mechanism protects neurons from death; such surprising neuron survival suggests that brain damage may be reversed for a much longer period than previously thought. The spirit of Lazarus does exist in brain cells.

The Genetic Turn-On

What about genes? Of course, genetic as well as prenatal influences help sculpt the brain. But experts do not think genes determine destiny. Other environmental factors, including diet, education, and lifestyle are also powerful determinants of mental functioning. "The genes are the bricks and mortar to build a brain. The environment is the architect," according to Christine Hohmann, neuroscientist at the Kennedy-Kriger Institute in Baltimore. As for worries about the aging brain, only about 30 percent of the characteristics of aging are genetically based; the rest—70 percent—are not, says leading aging researcher John Rowe at Mount Sinai Medical Center in New York. "People are largely responsible for their own old age."

Stress Can Damage Your Brain

The idea that hormones have an enormous impact on the brain is the subject of exciting new research. Scientists have long understood that circulating sex hormones shape the hippocampus, that part of the brain essential for remembering daily events and for certain forms of learning, during early brain development. Only recently have they come to realize that hormones, such as estrogen, and stress hormones, including cortisol, also help shape adult brains. This is good news–bad news.

Long-term chronic stress hormones are bad for the brain, say researchers. It's not just because such stress can make you uncomfortable, anxious, depressed, or fatigued. Recent research reveals that persistent stress can actually alter the very structure and functioning of your brain cells. The blunt truth: "Stress causes brain damage," says a leading brain authority, neuropsychiatrist Richard Restak, M.D. of the George Washington University School of Medicine and Health Sciences.

Stress triggers the "fight or flight syndrome," a primitive response that releases stress hormones (corticosteroids and adrenaline), mobilizing the body to save itself from danger, such as a roaring lion in the jungle. Today as then, short-lived stress may be good for brain functioning. The stress of taking a test, for example, can stimulate a burst of adrenaline that improves memory. But long-lasting, inappropriate stress triggered by everyday events, such as work frustration, traffic jams, and financial worries can wear your brain down, eroding important neuronal connections, eventually bringing on forgetfulness. Research suggests that chronic stress can actually shrink the hippocampus, the memory center of the brain.

Animal studies by renowned authority on stress and the brain Robert Sapolsky, professor of neuroscience at Stanford, show that a couple of weeks of exposure to elevated glucocorticoid levels cause neuronal dendrites to shrivel up, impairing message transmission. The good news: When glucocorticoid levels subside, dendrites can grow back. However, years of bathing in glucocorticoids from chronic stress may cause nerve cells responsible for memory to die. The loss looks for all the world like the death of neurons after a stroke or seizures, says prominent neuroscientist Dr. Bruce McEwen of Rockefeller University.

Stress also leads to the creation of free radical chemicals that can cause brain cells to atrophy and die.

Estrogen: The Memory Molecule

In contrast, many researchers believe the hormone estrogen is a potent preserver of memory in older women and possibly a partial antidote to Alzheimer's disease. Dr. David Snowdon, brain researcher at the University of Kentucky, calls estrogen "the number one candidate" for women seeking neuronal protection. "I recommend that older women take estrogen if they can," agrees Dr. Marilyn Albert, Harvard brain researcher.

Evidence of estrogen's brain benefits, notably for maintaining and restoring memory, has been accumulating for the last two decades. A recent breakthrough study by Barbara Sherwin at McGill University showed that women whose ovaries were removed, drying up supplies of estrogen, scored lower on cognitive tests, especially in verbal memory. Those who later got estrogen regained all their mental skills. Those denied estrogen in the double-blind trial did not.

New research also shows that estrogen rejuvenated memory centers in the brains of elderly women. When the women were taking estrogen, brain scans revealed "activation" patterns in short-term memory regions that resembled those in the brains of younger women. The dose was 1.25 milligrams daily.

Further, research at Columbia University found that postmenopausal women who had used estrogen replacement for ten years had one third the risk of developing Alzheimer's disease as women who never took it. Not a single woman who took estrogen replacement during the five year study developed Alzheimer's disease. Nationwide tests are underway to see if estrogen will delay or reverse mental deterioration in Alzheimer's patients.

How does estrogen work? Several ways, according to much research. It's known that estrogen increases the activity of neurotransmitters, notably acetylcholine, that are deeply involved in memory. Estrogen also stimulates the growth of dendrites and synapses in nerve cells, enhancing communication channels. Further, recent research identifies estrogen as a strong antioxidant that shields brain cells from destruction by free radical chemicals. Cell studies show that estrogen reduces the ability of brain cell toxins, such as glutamate and a protein called beta amyloid found in Alzheimer's brains, to generate destructive free radicals.

Use It or Lose It

One of the most novel avenues of brain research has produced astonishing evidence that the way you use your brain can alter its very form. Stimulating your brain intellectually and physically can actually cause measurable changes in its structure. Such activity can prod the brain to produce new connections between neurons and even create brand-new brain cells! That's what many scientists now say, based on very recent research. Unquestionably, it happens in laboratory rats, according to remarkable findings.

A research team headed by William T. Greenough, of the University of Illinois at Urbana-Champaign, raised rats in three different environments—alone in cages, two to a cage, and in a large playground cage with many young rats, toys, and treadmills—"a Disneyland for rats," in Dr. Greenough's words. He compared the complexity of their brain cells. What he found was startling. Within only four days of exposure to the "Disney wonderland of fun and games" the rats' brains went wild with new growth—the density of their synapses and the length of their dendrites increased profusely and rapidly. In short, the animals in the stimulating environment suddenly acquired more connections per nerve cell—more synapses—and a lush forest of dendrites. Their brains also grew new blood vessels to transport more blood and oxygen required to feed the rats' more active brain cells. Plus, the round bodies of the neurons grew bigger. Dr. Greenough put the rats through their paces in mazes and other tasks and found the stimulated rats performed better and were smarter.

Older rats put into the "rat wonderland" also grew more new connections between brain cells, compared with those left to languish in a restricted, dull environment—"cage potatoes," Dr. Greenough calls them. However, the brains of the old rats sprouted new connections more slowly than did the brains of young rats.

Dr. Greenough theorizes that the rats' stimulating lifestyle switched on genes in nerve cells, producing proteins that spurred the new growth of dendrites and synapses.

Also exciting are more recent studies by neuroscientist Fred Gage and colleagues at the Salk Institute for Biological Studies in La Jolla, California. They took newborn rats and put some in ordinary laboratory housing and others in an "enriched" environment with climbing tubes and running wheels, novel food, and lots of social interaction. Two months later, the "teenage" rats were subjected to brain examination, using a tracer drug to pinpoint new brain cells. According to Dr. Gage, the researchers counted every cell in the hippocampus of both sets of rats. The rats who grew up in ordinary digs had 270,000 neurons on each hemisphere of the hippocampus. Incredibly, the rats who grew up in the rollicking fun-and-games environment had an extra 50,000 brain cells in each side of their hippocampus. Thus, the stimulating environment added nearly twenty percent more brain cells, strategically placed in the memory and learning center of their brains!

Other tests on stimulated mice showed essentially the same startling increase in number of neurons and branching dendrites. Moreover, mice that lived in a stimulating environment were smarter, performing better on water maze tests of memory and learning than mice housed in spartan surroundings. Scientists explain that some neurons typically form in the brains of animals after birth, but usually die quickly. In the stimulated animals the newly formed cells mysteriously live on, increasing intellect. Janice Juraska, neuroscientist at the University of Illinois, calls such experiments "a unique demonstration of the power of the environment to sculpt the brain." The implications for young children are mind-boggling.

Educated Brains Are Stronger Brains

Why do women with college degrees live several years longer and retain better mental and physical abilities after age seventy-five than their less educated sisters? Why is Alzheimer's more apt to strike those who are less educated?

It's true that the better educated you are, the less likely you are to experience memory deterioration and dementia as you age. At first glance, this may seem extremely odd or more likely an indication that higher socioeconomic status or early avoidance of poverty and malnutrition convey special favors to the brain. Certainly, malnutrition influences brain functioning and, undeniably, genetics help define your upper limits of brain development.

But actually, nature's design is more egalitarian. Whether your brain emerges relatively unscathed in middle and old age depends much more on your own mental efforts than you may have imagined. The idea is that exerting your brain intellectually, starting in childhood, spurs brain cells to explode with new branches, creating millions of new connections, or synapses, between neurons. This means consistent mental stimulation actually builds more brain tissue, giving you a "bigger memory board," so you can think more quickly. It also means that you have built up a bigger surplus of brain cells to call on, should your brain run into trouble with a stroke, brain injury, or degenerative brain disease such as Alzheimer's.

Dr. David Snowdon, at the University of Kentucky's Sanders-Brown Center on Aging, heads a long-range study of elderly nuns who donated their brains after death for autopsy. Dr. Snowdon suspects, among other things, that the most highly educated nuns, signifying brain stimulation, have a larger cortex with more branches and connections. This, he believes, enables them to withstand even Alzheimer's disease with less evidence of mental devastation. "Nuns with the highest educational and intellectual life suffer least from symptoms of Alzheimer's," says Dr. Snowdon.

Unquestionably, scientists find a startling difference in the brain cells of laboratory rats raised in a stimulating environment. The neurons of stimulated rats are studded with extensive, long, and complex branches of dendrites; unstimulated rats have neurons with pathetically few short straggles of hairlike dendrites.

Arnold Scheibel, director of the Brain Research Institute at UCLA, credits evolution. He says the brain literally thrives on novelty in order to survive. "The brain stem has an area called the reticular formation. It's wired to respond selectively to the new and exotic. This was a survival mechanism when we were on the lookout for predators. Now, new challenges activate your reticular formation and stimulate the growth of dendrites. That's why people should not only remain active, but take up new pursuits."

In a word, if you have more brain matter in reserve, from a lifetime of using your brain, you are apt to decline intellectually at a far later age than someone who did not vigorously exercise his or her brain. As experts analogize, the brain is like a muscle—using it makes it grow and expand; disuse causes it to atrophy. Thus, education makes brains more resistant to deterioration and disease, because people who earn degrees tend to exercise their brains more, building a more lively, resilient, and complex brain.

"Learning switches on genes in nerve cells which in turn stimulates growth of dendrites and synapses."
—William T. Greenough, University of Illinois at Urbana-Champaign

Having more synapses, dendrites, and neurons also may slow brain impairment as you get older. The more of them you have, the more you must lose before you see signs of failing memory and other mental functions as you age. For example, much research shows that the more severe the dementia in Alzheimer's, the fewer the number of synapses between cells in the cerebral cortex, says brain researcher Robert Katzman, M.D., of the University of California, San Diego, School of Medicine. He also finds that people with more education are less likely to develop Alzheimer's, possibly because they use their brains more, keeping cells in shape. He conducted an epidemiological study in China, showing that less educated Chinese are four times more likely to die from dementias than better educated Chinese. Dr. Katzman suggests that getting more education may delay the onset of Alzheimer's symptoms by about five years.

Neurologist John Stirling Meyer and colleagues at Baylor College of Medicine in Houston studied 94 healthy people over age sixty-five for four years. Roughly one-third of the participants still had jobs; another third, although retired, stayed active mentally and physically, and the remaining third were relatively inactive. Subjects were given standard IQ and other neurological and psychological tests at the beginning of the study and at the end. At the start, everyone had normal scores on the tests. After four years, the inactive group scored lower on IQ tests and on tests measuring blood flow to their brains.

Exercise Expands Brains

A few years ago scientists were blown away by experiments showing that putting rats on treadmills induced their brain cells to produce a chemical "growth factor" that spurs growth of dendrites, thereby expanding communication networks. Most remarkable, the neuronal growth happened not only in parts of the brain that control motor function, but also in areas that control memory, reasoning, thinking, and learning, according to the research by Carl Cotman and colleagues at the University of California at Irvine. Exercise also increased blood flow to the brain. Dr. Cotman later found that older humans who exercised scored higher on tests of cognitive function than nonexercisers.

Remarkable new findings by Arthur Kramer of the University of Illinois at Urbana-Champaign further prove how exercise infuses new life into the brain. Dr. Kramer tested the cognitive functioning of 124 men and women, ages sixty to seventy-five, who never or rarely exercised. He put them on a three-times-a-week regimen of either aerobic exercise—a brisk one-hour walk—or yoga-type stretching. After six months, the walkers scored 25 percent higher than the stretchers on cognitive tests of "executive control" or "executive memory." The boost occurred in "higher" functions of decision-making, planning, scheduling, ability to quickly switch tasks, look up and remember phone numbers—skills essential for independent living, yet the first to decline as you get older. Dr. Kramer believes aerobic exercise pumps more blood to the brain's frontal cortex that controls executive functions.

Other researchers find that exercise raises levels of free-radical fighters to protect brain cells and that activity of any type improves mood.

"Simply running a few days a week increases brain proteins, and that helps protect nerve cells from injury, cells known to be associated with cognition." —Carl Cotman, University of California at Irvine

Truly we have entered a new miracle age of the brain, bursting with the promise of unprecedented emotional and intellectual fulfillment. Scientists for the first time in history are beginning to comprehend the brain's awesome "plasticity"—its stunning ability to continually reinvent itself. All of us alive today are the beneficiaries of this new knowledge.

PART 2

WHAT TO EAT FOR A MIRACLE BRAIN

The Ancient Diet Your Brain Most Craves

Nature's grand design for your brain's nutrient needs was laid out a few million years ago. It's still the best guide to brain-building foods.

Imagine that you were entrusted with designing a prototype of the human brain a few million years ago. Logically, its form would be greatly dictated by the available sustenance to keep it alive and functioning perfectly. Indeed, the fuel should be in absolute harmony with the biomechanics of the brain. Since the brain is an organic structure, what you feed it, in fact, would actually determine its final architecture and function, and would also determine what it should be fed for the rest of time.

You would not expect an electric engine to run on gasoline; it's just as foolish to expect your brain to run smoothly on fuel at odds with its basic nature.

To get your brain in sync with your highest potential, it's important to feed it a diet true to its ancient genetic origins—the diet that nourished brains during our evolutionary infancy when our Paleolithic ancestors foraged for plants and fished and hunted, thousands of years before the cultivation of grains and the domestication of animals and a time-warp away from the establishment of fast-food chains, processed foods, and supermarkets.

During its formative period over the past three million years the human brain grew and changed; its very architecture and intricate wiring were dictated by the foods available at the time. Its cells thrived on the type of fats most abundant and compatible. It set up communication systems based on enzymes made from nutrients in fruits, nuts, vegetables, and other wild plants. It organized protective systems for brain cells based on natural antioxidants to help ensure its oxygen-based survival. It made genes to control life-processes from nutrient building blocks delivered by the ancient diet. Thus, the genetic makeup and daily diet of the body formed a perfect union, and the result was a brain that functioned as nature designed.

Today, our diet and our brain's demands are a colossal mismatch. Our genes have not changed significantly for several million years, but our diet has changed radically within the last fifty years.

Small wonder, then, that our brains frequently malfunction, sending us into abnormal states of depression, psychosis, memory decline, lowered intelligence, and dementia. It seems clear that sometimes, in evolutionary terms, our brains are running on empty, because our modern diets are so incongruent with our genetic makeup. Much of the stuff we feed our brains is completely foreign to our genes. Our brain craves nutrients based on its evolutionary memory, common foods of forty thousand years ago—we feed it stuff that didn't exist even forty years ago. Our brains yearn for the nutrients in a Stone Age diet. We feed them McDonald's and Mazola corn oil. It's hard to imagine the mighty famine this must unleash inside the landscape of the brain.

> **BOTTOM LINE:** *The essence—the biochemistry and physiology—of our brains is fine-tuned to a long-lost diet that existed in prehistoric days.*
>
> *"The largely new dietary pattern adopted since the invention of agriculture, and especially within the past one hundred years, appears to go beyond what our genes can tolerate."* —S. Boyd Eaton, M.D., Emory University, *The Paleolithic Prescription*

From Wild Greens to Big Macs

At least a hundred thousand generations of our ancestors survived on the Stone Age foods of hunters and gatherers— wild game, wild greens, fruits, berries, and roots. Then about ten thousand years ago the world was rocked by an historical event. The agricultural revolution rapidly swept the earth. Most scholars say it was a boon for humankind, leading to new organizations, stable social structures and governments, cities, and a burst of human achievement. However, the infusion of foreign foods into the body and brain most certainly delivered a biological jolt, still unresolved and troublesome. Humans turned to cultivating grains, making breads, and keeping herds of animals, including those that gave milk and provided eggs. Two new food groups—cereals, bread, and grains; and dairy products—joined the two ancient food groups—fruits and vegetables; meats and fish. Most of the human race was now existing primarily on a steady supply of cultivated foods with which the body had little history. The brain was required to incorporate nutrients that were not an integral part of its origins or genetic makeup.

This dietary pattern existed for about five hundred generations, until the twentieth century, when, spurred by modern industrialization, another dietary upheaval occurred: the advent of processed and fast foods, which have been around on a massive scale for less than three generations—a mere fifty to sixty years. It's doubtful that our brains can adapt to such a radically different diet in such an infinitesimally short evolutionary time without going a little haywire.

It's also unthinkable that we can turn back time to totally embrace a Stone Age diet, but it's smart to try to make our modern diets more compatible with foods medical anthropologists tell us our cells need historically to function at peak power.

Here's the Diet That Formed Our Brains

Basically, Stone Age humans foraged for wild plants—fruits, berries, roots, legumes, nuts—and hunted for wild game and seafood. They ate virtually none of the grains that dominates our diets. Nor did they have domesticated animals for dairy products. This diet was the norm for a couple million years. Our modern diet, in evolutionary terms, is quite novel, merely an instant in human history.

> **ALARMING FACT:** We have departed so far from Stone-Age eating that 55 percent of the American diet is made up of "new foods," not consumed by our ancient ancestors.

STONE-AGE DIET:
65% Fruits, vegetables, nuts, legumes, honey
35% Lean game, wild fowl, eggs, fish, shellfish

AMERICAN DIET:
55% "new" foods: Cereal, grains, milk, milk products, sugar, sweeteners, separated fats, alcohol.
28% Fatty meat, poultry, eggs, fish, shellfish
17% Fruits, vegetables, legumes, nuts

A Guide to Our Ancient Brain-Boosting Diet

According to "evolutionary nutritionist" Dr. Boyd Eaton, of Emory University in Atlanta and co-author of *The Paleolithic Prescription*, here's what to eat and not eat to get more of the nutrients that sculpted our brains.

- Fruits and vegetables: Overwhelmingly, the primary staples among our Stone-Age ancestors were fruits and vegetables, notably berries and other fruits. They ate three times more of a wider variety of fruits and vegetables than we do. Along with nuts and legumes, fruits and vegetables provided a startling 65 percent of daily calories and about 100 grams of fiber a day—ten times our average intake. Fruits and vegetables supplied loads of vitamins, minerals, and antioxidants in amounts people now get only through supplements, says Dr. Eaton.

- Seafood galore: One of the most critical distinctions between a Stone-Age and modern diet is the right balance of omega-6 fats to brain-enhancing omega-3 fish-type fats. The Paleolithic ratio was one part omega-6 fat to one part omega-3 (or four to one, at most), which promoted smooth brain functioning. Today the omega-6s in the form of corn oils, margarines, and baked goods outstrip fish-type omega-3s by fifteen or twenty to one. It's a sickening situation for cells, particularly brain cells, which simply malfunction or shut down if omega-3 fat is scarce and omega-6 is overwhelming. Thus, the only way to reinstate a brain-enhancing Stone-Age type diet is to eat fatty fish, notably fatty salmon, sardines, mackerel, and herring, and/or take fish oil capsules and restrict omega 6s.

- Only lean meat: Our Stone-Age ancestors ate 37 percent of their calories in protein—two to three times that recommended today, says Dr. Eaton. The difference: Most protein came from lean wild game and fish, as well as from plants. Wild game that fed our early evolutionary selves was only 4.3 percent fat, compared with 25 to 30 percent fat in today's major meat sources. Further, wild game was a source of all-important omega-3, essential for brain development. Wild game fat contains 2.5 percent EPA omega-3. It is virtually nonexistent in domesticated beef.

  Unlike Stone-Age meats, modern red meat is full of hazardous saturated fats. Our ancestors ate only 6 percent of calories in such animal fat, about half as much as we do. White meat poultry, without skin, is a good Stone-Age meat equivalent, low in fat and a good source of protein.

- Nuts and legumes: Unfortunately, nuts have a bad rap because of their fat; but nuts are an "original" food, with fats attuned to our genes. Our Stone-Age ancestors ate all kinds of tree nuts as well as peanuts and other legumes (dried beans). Nuts and legumes also supply high-grade vegetable protein, rich in Stone-Age diets. A modern drawback: Canned dried beans and salted nuts are high in sodium which is incompatible with Stone-Age genes. To avoid high sodium, cook your own beans without salt, thoroughly rinse canned beans to remove sodium, and buy unsalted nuts.

- Cereals, pasta, bread: Cultivated grain-based foods are "new," for our brains, a product of the ten-thousand-year-old Agricultural Revolution. Virtually absent in Stone-Age diets, grains had no part in fashioning our genes. Yet they are a major part of modern diets. Grains may not be harmful in themselves, says Dr. Eaton, but he fears they replace all-important fruits and vegetables, which have been staples in our diets for millions of years, "whereas grains have been staples for only a relatively few millennia." Other researchers note that grains, notably wheat, can trigger subtle allergic reactions in many people, prompting headaches and depression, as well as arthritis and gastrointestinal problems, suggesting a genetic disharmony.

- Dairy foods: Our Stone-Age ancestors did not drink milk or use dairy products because they did not keep domesticated animals. Such milk products may screw up body functioning by adding high burdens of saturated fats and discordant proteins. We are the only mammals that continue to use milk products past the weaning stage, points out Dr. Eaton. To mimic a Stone-Age diet, you should restrict milk, butter, cheese, and other dairy products. For some people, dairy foods are clearly gene-incompatible, because they lack the enzymes needed to digest milk. Cow's milk is also a common cause of allergies.

- Sugar: Our remote ancestors used honey and fruits as sweeteners. Today, our main sweet is about 120 pounds of refined sugar a year. Actually, we eat about the same percentage of carbohydrates as our Stone-Age ancestors. But virtually all their carbos came from nutrient-rich fruits and vegetables. A mere one-quarter of ours come from fruits and vegetables. Most of our carbos are simple "empty calorie" sugar. How this unnatural overload of sugar affects our genes and our brains is unclear, but is apt to be quite detrimental. For sure, it drives up blood levels of insulin, glucose, and triglycerides, with dire implications for stroke and brain dysfunction.

- Processed oils: Our recent upsurge in consumption of processed vegetable oils and shortenings burdens our brains with unfamiliar types of fat. Stone-Age ancestors ate only fat in foods, not as separated oils, and consumed about 22 percent in fat calories compared with our 35 percent. An overload of polyunsaturated fats, including hydrogenated and trans fats, triggers cell malfunction that is bad for the brain. Some oils are more compatible with brain needs: canola oil, olive oil, flaxseed oil.

- Potassium and sodium: The most striking way to mimic a Stone-Age diet is to eat far more potassium than sodium. Our Stone-Age ancestors got 7000 milligrams of potassium daily, mainly in fruits and vegetables, and a mere 600 milligrams of sodium, compared with our paltry 2500 milligrams of potassium, and whopping 4000 milligrams of sodium. Humans are the only free-living mammals that eat more sodium than potassium, says Dr. Eaton. And we pay a high price in our death and disability toll from high blood pressure and strokes.

FACT: Our Stone-Age ancestors ate more calories (3000 a day) than we do (2000–2500) but burned more off in physical activity.

FACT: Stone-Age humans typically took in one and a half to five times more vitamins and minerals than we do today in food, far exceeding our minimum recommended standards.

TEN WAYS TO FEED YOUR BRAIN
WHAT IT REALLY WANTS

1. Make fruits and vegetables the major part of your diet.
2. Eat poultry without skin, or very lean meats and game.
3. Eat dried beans—legumes of all kinds, including peanuts, preferably unsalted.
4. Eat nuts, notably walnuts and almonds.
5. Eat fatty fish (salmon, sardines, mackerel), shell-fish.
6. Restrict omega-6 fats (especially corn oil), hydrogenated vegetable oils, and trans fatty acids.
7. Restrict sugar and sodium.
8. Restrict processed foods.
9. Take vitamin-mineral supplements, because it is impossible to totally imitate a nutrient-rich Stone-Age diet without a boost from supplements.
10. Take fish oil capsules, especially if you don't eat fish several times a week.

BOTTOM LINE: *The closer you get to the original food source, the closer you are to the brain-boosting diet designed by your brain's ancient architects.*

How Fat Can Make and Break Your Brain

Nothing you put in your mouth is as agreeable or disagreeable to the intricate structures of your brain cells as fat. Your brain is the body's fattiest organ—60 percent is made up of lipids (various types of fatlike substances). The chemistry of that fat can profoundly influence the very architecture of your brain cells, the profusion or scarcity of all-important dendrites and synapses—the linchpins of intelligence, learning, memory, attention, concentration, and mood. Fat molecules also help determine how much of which type neurotransmitters brain cells make and release—whether they switch on genes and hormones that make you feel good or bad or harm or benefit your brain.

Bad Fat, Brain Breakdown

Unless you feed your brain its required quota of the right fat and withhold the bad fats, it can become inefficient and possibly dysfunctional. There is no question about it. Denied the right fat molecules and flooded with the bad ones, your cerebral tissue may become partly starved—not a pretty picture. The outer membranes of your brain cells may stiffen and shrivel; the dendritic tentacles that reach out to form patterns of communication with other cells may become stunted; the rich chemical flood of neuro-transmitters may dry up or become short-circuited, unable to gain entry to neurons and carry messages from neuron to neuron. It is a mess that nature never intended. Yet, that is the state of many people's brains.

Scientists used to think that eating fat had virtually no impact on the functioning of adult brains—that it was essential only to the developing brains of infants and children. Dogma held that the one chance to build a great brain ended by adolescence because by that age the brain was fixed and unchangeable, incapable of further growth. Now we know that neurons can continue to grow and expand at all ages, even into old age. Such growth requires supplies of fatty acids. Thus, the fat you eat throughout life is constantly molding your brain. It's an exciting but sobering thought, considering the low-quality fat most of us feed our brain cells.

> *Bottom line: The type fat you put in your brain from birth to death is one of the most critical decisions you can ever make for the good or detriment of your brain.*

The Fat That Stunts Your Brain

Here's something to keep in mind the next time you and/or your kids go to a fast food restaurant for hamburgers, milk shakes, and fries or for a pizza loaded with fatty cheese: Such saturated fat may actually stunt the growth of your brain cells.

Compelling research in small laboratory animals shows that the type of fat in the diet can actually change not just the function of brain cells, but their very shape—their morphology. In short, the fat you eat can change the configuration of your brain cells, for better or worse.

Researchers have known for more than a decade that

GOOD AND BAD BRAIN FATS AT A GLANCE

BRAIN BOOSTING FATS:

- DHA: The top gun omega-3 type brain fat. You get it from eating seafood, or taking supplements.
- EPA: The other high potency omega-3 brain fat comes from eating fish or taking fish oil.
- Linolenic acid: The short-chain omega-3s that your body must transform to long-chain omega-3s to be beneficial to your brain. You get it in green leafy vegetables, nuts, and flaxseed.
- Monounsaturated fat, as in olive oil: Contains some antioxidants, does not increase vascular threats, and has been found to benefit memory.

BRAIN-BUSTING FATS:

- Saturated animal fat: Meat, whole milk, butter, cheese.
- Hydrogenated vegetable oils: Margarine, mayonnaise, processed foods. Check the label.
- Trans fatty acids: Margarine, processed foods, fried fast foods, such as french fries.
- Overloads of omega-6 vegetable oils: Processed foods; vegetable oils such as corn, safflower, and sunflower oils.

saturated fat does something awful to mammalian brains. Laboratory animals fed lots of saturated lard don't learn as quickly or perform as well on a wide spectrum of memory tests, including finding their way out of mazes, as do animals fed polyunsaturated soybean oil. Indeed, lard-fed animals consistently display impaired short and long-term spatial memory, resulting in learning and memory dysfunction on a wide range of tasks and functions involving several regions of the brain, as well as neurotransmitters. This indicates that dietary fat has sweeping effects on brain function and helps manipulate extremely complex cognitive behavior in animals, says University of Toronto professor Carol E. Greenwood, Ph.D., a pioneering researcher in the effects of fat on the brain.

The major villain is saturated fat; it predictably causes major detrimental effects on memory and learning; monounsaturated fat (olive oil) may be beneficial to memory, and polyunsaturated fat may be detrimental or beneficial, depending on the type. The more saturated fats animals eat, the more severe their brain and memory malfunction. Dr. Greenwood demonstrated that rats' learning curves dropped in direct proportion to the amount of saturated fat they ate. On a diet of ten percent saturated fat, the animals learned virtually nothing!

FACT: When you feed animals a high saturated fat diet, they don't learn as rapidly.

Further, the harmful effects of saturated fat on the brain seem to be cumulative. The more years you consistently eat a high animal fat diet, the more severe the risk of "dumbing down." In fact, it appears the brain over time begins to adapt to a high animal fat diet, resulting in impaired learning. Thus, the danger comes from a long-time pattern of a high saturated fat diet. A periodic splurge of a hot fudge sundae or cream pie is not likely to be detrimental in the long run, says Dr. Greenwood. Moreover, animal studies suggest that a consistent high saturated fat diet seems to somehow exert a direct toxic antilearning effect on brain cells regardless of the other types of fat you eat. In other words, the danger comes from the saturated fat itself, not just an imbalance or lack of other beneficial fats.

More frightening, the amount of saturated fat needed to produce memory impairment in animals is comparable to the amount Americans typically eat! It's logical then that such high animal fat diets may be subtle inducers of poor learning in young people and of accelerated age-related memory loss in adults. Studies also find high saturated fat associated with degenerative brain diseases, notably Parkinson's disease. A study by Richard Mayeux and colleagues at Columbia University showed that people over age sixty-five who ate the most animal fat were *five times* more apt to develop Parkinson's than those who ate the least animal fat.

It's not exactly clear how saturated fat messes up brain cells. There are many theories, involving changes in composition of cell membranes; electrical activity of neurotransmitters, notably serotonin; manipulation of enzymes; attacks by free radicals; decreased insulin sensitivity (increase in insulin resistance); and the uptake and utilization of glucose, a powerful substance in the brain.

But now comes another astonishing discovery showing that saturated fat may literally strangle brain cells. Groundbreaking new research by Patricia Wainwright and colleagues in the Department of Health Studies, Gerontology, and Psychology at the University of Waterloo in Ontario, Canada, finds that saturated fat does more than influence the brain cell's function; such fat can actually alter the morphology, or shape, of the brain cells themselves! Visual examinations of brain cells retrieved after death from animals fed lots of saturated fat as fetuses and for eight weeks after birth reveal neurons that are stunted! Analyses of the gray matter of the fat-fed animals showed fewer and shorter dendrites with fewer of the branches needed to reach out to send and receive messages. In addition to having runted dendrites, the high-saturated-fat-fed mice had generally lighter-weight brains, as well as smaller bodies.

Dr. Greenwood explains that stunted dendrites can cripple memory, because physical changes actually take place in brain cells during memory and learning. "During periods of memory when someone is learning," she says, "we see an expansion of dendrites; thus, dendritic expansion seems to be necessary in terms of memory function. Now if high-saturated-fat diets are limiting the ability of the neuron to expand during memory processes, it may partly explain why animals eating high fat diets have such poor memory performance. Scientifically, it's a very important finding, revealing a possible new way saturated fat influences brain functioning."

Discovering the Enemy

Recently many scientists have rallied around another new theory, proposing that saturated fat degrades memory and learning by affecting the hormone insulin. Both animals and humans who eat lots of saturated fat tend to develop insulin resistance. This means insulin becomes less "sensitive" and less efficient at handling blood glucose. The result: disturbances of glucose utilization throughout the body, including the brain, and possibly cognitive impairment. For example, diabetics typically have high blood glucose and poorly functioning insulin. It's also increasingly recognized that persons with both insulin-dependent diabetes (Type I) and non-insulin-dependent diabetes (Type 2) tend to develop various types of cognitive impairment, including memory problems.

Researchers increasingly believe, says Dr. Greenwood, that the major underlying reason saturated fat harms the brain is that it predisposes a person to insulin resistance, a condition that precedes and accompanies diabetes, and is the root of the memory problems. "What we may be seeing in animals and humans who eat a lot of fat is insulin resistance or a prediabetic state," she says, "leading to memory impairment."

Now that's scary. So-called insulin resistance is almost epidemic in the United States and worsening. Who has it? The vast majority of adults with diabetes or impaired glucose tolerance, about half of everyone with high blood pressure, and about one-fourth of Americans who are considered healthy, says Stanford University's Gerald M. Reaven, M.D., a leading expert in diabetes. That suggests that nearly one hundred million Americans could be suffering from insulin-resistance-related memory problems! Millions of us could be having this memory loss and not even know it.

"That's right," says Dr. Greenberg. If the evidence proves out as she thinks it will, she agrees that "it's scary." On the other hand, she points to the bright side: "It's reversible. It's not permanent damage." When diabetes, hence insulin and glucose, is controlled by drugs, diet, weight loss, or other remedies, memory and learning ability usually return to normal, she says. Thus, similar lifestyle changes can prevent or reverse insulin resistance, this "prediabetic state" that threatens your brain, memory, and intellectual functioning.

BOTTOM LINE: *A high animal fat diet may help push you into a prediabetic or diabetic state, causing insulin and glucose disturbances that mess up your brain and memory.*

"I would say that any lifestyle factor that would lead to the development of insulin resistance may contribute to memory decline." —Dr. Carol Greenwood, University of Toronto

"There are more and more insulin-resistant people every day because the population is getting fatter and older." —Judith Hallfrisch, U.S. Department of Agriculture's Human Nutrition Research Center in Beltsville, Maryland

Alarming Epidemic in Children

Among the distressing new findings: Doctors for the first time are seeing skyrocketing rates of insulin resistance and Type 2 diabetes—an adult disease—in *children, notably obese children*. According to a 1999 study, every single one of twenty-one overweight children, ages ten to seventeen, had characteristic signs of insulin resistance, reported endocrinologist Robin Goland, Columbia Presbyterian Medical Center in New York. This is an alarming change. Insulin resistance and Type 2 (adult-onset) diabetes traditionally strike adults past forty and are rare in children.

Only five to ten years ago, virtually all childhood diabetes was Type 1—insulin-dependent—diabetes usually starting around age twelve and unrelated to obesity, says Dr. Goland. Now about twenty percent of new cases of diabetes in children and adolescents are the "adult" type, related to overweight, insulin resistance, and a high-fat diet. The implications are disturbing. It suggests that serious diabetic "complications," including memory problems and dulled mental functioning, as well as heart disease, might be accelerated in these children, showing up at ages twenty to thirty instead of in old age, say experts. "The situation is absolutely shocking," says Jennie Brand-Miller, an associate professor of nutrition specializing in blood glucose research at the University of Sydney in Australia.

Even more ominous is the prospect that our growing epidemic of insulin resistance is causing memory decline in large numbers of unsuspecting persons who silently accept it as a consequence of "normal aging." For several years scientists have known that insulin resistance promotes high blood pressure, high triglycerides, low good HDL cholesterol and clogged arteries, all of which can indirectly promote brain damage and compromise mental functioning. Now there's reason to think this spreading health menace also directly harms the brain and memory.

Animal fat is not the only route to insulin resistance. A high carbohydrate diet, especially one high in quickly digested carbos with a "high glycemic index," is also a prime culprit (see page 125); and too much animal protein can also contribute to insulin resistance. There's also evidence that eating fish oil helps defeat insulin resistance by making fatty membranes more "fluid." Such fluid membranes have greater numbers of and more responsive insulin receptors, heightening their sensitivity to insulin, says Artemis P. Simopoulos, M.D., president of The Center for Genetics, Nutrition and Health and author of a book on fish oil called *The Omega Plan*.

Still, a major way to avoid or overcome insulin resistance that may cause glucose and brain malfunction is to stop eating a high saturated fat diet. That gives your brain a chance to recover. Since it takes years for excessive saturated fat to foster a sluggish brain, it's likely to "take time after you stop eating a high saturated fat diet before you see benefits," as glucose and insulin functioning improve, says Dr. Greenwood.

It's obviously better not to spend a large part of your life on a high-saturated fat regimen, especially in the early years. It's frightening to contemplate what such diets are doing to our children's formative brains, as well as to aging ones. Understanding that animal fat does not just lead to heart disease years down the road, but may also degrade your mental faculties earlier in life—contributing to a form of "presenility"—should be more powerful at deterring animal fat consumption than traditional warnings. The hopeful news is reversibility: Your brain is apt to bounce back when no longer subjected to high-fat abuse, says Dr. Greenwood.

Processed Oil as Brain Buster

There is another alarming way fat can harm your brain: overeating one type fat and skimping on another type, thus ignoring evolutionary wisdom. Most Americans are filling their brain cells full of the wrong kind of fat and ignoring the right type fat, creating a very destructive imbalance. Among so-called polyunsaturated fatty acids, there are two basic types of fat, one called omega-6 fat and the other omega-3 fat. They have distinctly different chemical make-ups. During prehistoric days when our brains evolved, our ancestors ate equal amounts of omega-3 and omega-6. Omega-3 is found in seafood; our bodies also made some from other fatty acids found in nuts, greens, and lean meat. The omega-6s at that time came mostly from fruits and vegetables, nuts and legumes. (Today omega-6s come primarily from processed vegetable oils.)

This ideal fat ratio prevailed for about four million years until the 1800s. The Industrial Revolution brought drastic changes, including the processing of high omega-6 vegetable oils. Wild, lean game was replaced with high-fat cattle and pigs. In the last one hundred and fifty years, intakes of saturated fat and omega-6s skyrocketed while consumption of omega-3s plunged to pathetic lows. Today,

Americans, feasting on processed oil and Big Macs, eat from fifteen to twenty times more omega-6 fats than omega-3 fats. This ratio is wildly out of sync with our genetic origins, and we are paying a high price in accelerated aging and sky-high rates of chronic disease.

Your brain, because it is made up mostly of fat—fat you feed it—is the prime target of this dangerous fat imbalance. Excesses of bad fats and shortages of good fats can eventually lead to brain cell dysfunction and death, deteriorating mental faculties in people of all ages, notably in the young and the old.

> **ALARMING FACT:** Even though we eat a lot of fat, it is not the right type for optimal brain functioning. Americans typically eat fifteen times more potentially brain-destructive type oils than we do brain-building omega-3 fish-type fats.

When Bad Omega-6s Rule Your Brain

It's amazing how the landscape of your brain changes when you eat too much polyunsaturated fat, chemically classified as omega-6s. Your brain literally becomes a battlefield where omega-3 fatty acids (in fish) and omega-6s (in vegetable oils and dressings) fight for control of your cells. And because of their huge numbers, due to our prodigious intakes, the omega-6s usually win, establishing tyrannical rule over neuronal activity. These constant omega-6 victories create havoc in the brain.

One of the most fearful potential consequences of omega-6 dominance in brain cells is persistent inflammation of brain tissue. Such inflammation can injure cerebral blood vessels, set up processes that kill brain cells, warp nerve cell membranes disrupting normal functioning, interfere with neuronal message transmission, and promote strokes, Alzheimer's disease, and probably all degenerative brain diseases. In new 1999 findings, evidence of chronic inflammation increased the odds of thromboembolic stroke by nearly 500 percent in a large group of men observed for twenty years as part of the Honolulu Heart Study.

Inflammation: The New Menace

Scientists now suspect chronic low-level inflammation may underlie much diverse neurological damage, including Alzheimer's disease. This discovery may help explain many odd facts: why people who take anti-inflammatory drugs, as for arthritis, have low rates of Alzheimer's and slower mental decline (more than twenty studies show this to be true); why fish oil, an anti-inflammatory substance, protects against brain damage and can alleviate depression; why aspirin, which fights inflammation, may reduce the risk of cerebrovascular disease in general and ischemic (blood clot) strokes in particular; why certain antioxidants that have anti-inflammatory activity, such as vitamin E and C, appear to protect against brain cell death and deterioration; and even why cholesterol-lowering statin drugs help ward off strokes and heart attacks. New research finds they are a potent anti-inflammatory.

Inflammation is a newly recognized enemy underlying gradual brain destruction, contributing to strokes, mood disorders, schizophrenia, and neurodegenerative diseases such as Alzheimer's, as well as "normal" mental decline.

Knowing that inflammation is in a sense a slow-acting nerve toxin, why would anyone want to regularly flood brain cells with the fuel to ignite inflammatory agents? They probably wouldn't. But then most people don't know that omega-6-type fat is such a fuel. It is scientifically well established that omega-6 fatty acids tend to be extremely pro-inflammatory.

It is a complex process, but essentially here's how it happens: When fats are metabolized (broken down for use), they spew off byproducts, some benign, some harmful, depending on the type fat. The metabolism of omega-6s sets off ferocious fireworks of incendiary byproducts of hormonelike substances known as eicosanoids—including prostaglandins, leukotrienes, and cytokines—as well as free-radical chemicals, all of which can trigger inflammation. For example, researchers consistently detect high levels of one type of pro-inflammatory prostaglandin—a hormone-like substance—in the brains of Alzheimer's patients, but not in the brains of nondemented elderly people. Dr. K.N. Prasad and colleagues at the University of Colorado Health Sciences Center in Denver have branded specific prostaglandins as "neurotoxins" because they kill brain cells. Such discoveries cause researchers to believe that the activation of such inflammatory mechanisms causes the degeneration of brain cells.

Pouring omega–6 fats into brain cells lights a fire throughout the brain that may end in nerve cell destruction.

One of the most frightening pro-inflammatory agents produced by the conversion of omega-6-type fat in cells is a chemical called arachidonic acid. Under certain circumstances it is deeply involved in nerve cell death. Besides spawning inflammatory eicosanoids and super-awful free-radical chemicals, arachidonic acid also can stimulate production of glutamate, a neurotransmitter, which is a natural-born cell killer. Recent research incriminates glutamate as the primary initiator of the execution of neurons, involved in brain damage from aging and strokes as well as degenerative brain diseases, including Alzheimer's.

By unleashing the fury of glutamate in cells, arachidonic acid triggers a cascade of molecular events ending in cells' actually being "excited" to death. Excessive glutamate provokes neurons to fire over and over, until they are exhausted. In so doing, a steady stream of free radicals is created and cellular calcium regulation gets so screwed up, levels build up inside neurons to toxic levels. At this point the nerve cell may become so dysfunctional, it issues an order to self-destruct. The cellular obituary lists as cause of death a process called "excitotoxicity." This "excitotoxicity" is thought to be one reason nerve cells die in Alzheimer's disease. If at any point this process can be interrupted, the neuron may survive. There are many possibilities for rescue—taking antioxidant supplements and anti-inflammatory drugs, even aspirin, for example. Another one is to stop eating so many omega-6s, thereby preventing oversupplies of toxic arachidonic acid from flooding brain cells. (For foods with the most omega-6s, see page 66.) Eating more omega-3 fish oil also helps defuse the "excitotoxic" brain damage, research shows.

You could also save your brain from excessive production of arachidonic acid and other agents of destruction in the first place by turning down inflammatory processes. Such inflammation was probably rare in ancient brains because of the proper balance of omega-6 fatty acids to omega-3 fatty acids. If you have enough omega-3s in brain cells, they can neutralize the ill effects of omega-6s. Thus, sending in forces of omega-3 molecules by eating fatty fish can help cool the fires kindled by omega-6s and curtail potential brain damage.

Omega-3 fats, in a word, help curtail the damage omega-6 fats can inflict on your brain cells, including the "excitotoxicity" process researchers believe is implicated in brain degeneration. Perhaps that's why people with lower levels of omega-3 fatty acids, particularly the fraction called DHA which is most active in nerve cells, are more apt to develop Alzheimer's disease.

So spectacular are the newly discovered brain benefits of eating omega-3 fish oil that the next chapter is devoted entirely to that amazing new research.

More Omega-6 Fat, More Memory Loss

Inferior brain functioning in humans who overeat omega-6 fats is not theoretical; it has been documented. Research shows that older people with high omega-6 diets have poorer mental functioning and more memory loss.

In a large Dutch study (the Zutphen Elderly Study) researchers analyzed the diets of some 1300 men, ages sixty-four to eighty-four. The men also took standard tests to assess their intellectual functioning. Clearly, men who ate the most omega-6 fat, primarily in margarines, baking fats, and sauces, had a 75 percent higher risk of cognitive impairment, including memory loss, than those who ate the least omega-6 fats. The intellectual decline of a smaller group of the men was measured over a three-year period. Those who ate the most omega-6 fats were 250 percent more apt to show signs of mental deterioration during that time than those who ate the least. Not surprisingly, eating fish proved to be an antagonist to mental decline. Eating more fish, a mere extra ounce a week, cut the men's risk of cognitive decline by 55 percent.

What's critical to the brain is not just the total amounts of omega-6 and omega-3 fatty acids you eat, but the relative amounts of each, or the ratio. In fact, the ratio is *the critical factor* that determines how well information is transmitted from neuron to neuron, according to research by prominent Israeli psychologist Shlomo Yehuda, at Bar-Ilan University in Ramat Gan.

BOTTOM LINE: *Don't let omega-6 fats dominate your brain cells. They dispatch assassins that cripple and kill your brain cells, leaving your mental capacities diminished. The solution: Cut back on omega-6 fats and eat more omega-3 fish oil fats.*

VEGETABLE OILS: NEW KILLERS IN JAPAN

The people of Okinawa, a region of islands in Japan, fifty years ago boasted the greatest longevity in the world. No longer. During the military occupation by the United States after World War II until 1972, their diet rapidly became more Westernized, changing to include more omega-6-type edible oils and less fish. Consequently, their reign as the champions of longevity also ended, say authorities. By 1990, longevity among Okinawan males had plunged to fifth among all regions of Japan; that year the death rates for Okinawan males under age fifty were the highest of any place in Japan. In a recent analysis, Japanese researchers attributed the fall in longevity to the "rapid Westernization" of the diet, mainly the switch to a high omega-6, low omega-3 diet, typical in Western nations. Obviously, this fatty imbalance that favors an abundance of omega-6 and a deficiency of omega-3 is not conducive to extending life, but to promoting premature death, they concluded.

How Much Is Too Much?

In a perfect ancient world, you would eat no more than one molecule of omega-6 fatty acid for every one molecule of omega-3 fatty acid for good brain functioning. But some authorities today suggest you can achieve excellent brain functioning by restricting omega-6 fatty acids to four molecules per every one molecule of omega-3 fatty acids or a ratio of four to one. Since most Americans now eat fifteen to twenty molecules of omega-6s to one molecule of omega-3, a four to one ratio is a sizable reduction, and can have profound benefits for the brain. Israel's Dr. Yehuda calls it the "optimal" ratio. In laboratory animals he has found that this four to one ratio vastly improved learning, improved sleep, reduced seizures, and even reversed to a large extent learning problems induced by nerve cell toxins.

Even minor changes can help rescue your brain from fatty acid imbalance. William Lands, Ph.D., a world-renowned authority on fish oil at the National Institutes of Health, says frequently substituting fatty fish, such as salmon or sardines, for meat and shunning omega-6 corn oils and most other salad dressings restores fat balance in cells, including neurons, to the desirable one-to-one ratio of our ancient ancestors.

Dr. Lands was one of a group of international experts who recently made first-of-a-kind recommendations for "adequate" intakes of omega-6s and omega-3s. Here are the daily amounts if you eat 2,000 calories a day: 4.4 grams of omega-6s; .65 grams or 650 milligrams of long-chain omega-3s in seafood, and 2.2 grams of short-chain omega-3s in walnuts and greens. Dr. Lands figures that eating those quotas of fatty acids would end up in the cells as a perfect balance of 50:50—one molecule of omega-6 for one molecule of omega-3—needed for regulation of cell functioning and suppression of destructive inflammatory agents.

However, it's somewhat startling to learn how quickly you can gobble up four grams of omega-6s. It's the amount in a mere *half tablespoon* of soybean or corn oil. Just to give you an idea of our excessive use, even that small daily amount, says Dr. Lands, is far more than the cells really need to function optimally. Most Americans already have large amounts of omega-6s stored in their fatty tissue—enough to last at least a year or more. A shortage of omega-6s is almost unimaginable, considering the enormous quantities we eat.

To Dr. Lands, who for thirty years has warned of the toxicity of omega-6 fats, salad dressings are the most destructive source. "Everybody should eat less salad oils all around," he says, especially ones made with corn oil and soybean oil. Best choices: olive oil and canola oils with fairly low amounts of omega-6s; canola oil also has high omega-3s. And there's some evidence olive oil specifically protects the brain.

Olive Oil Saves Memory

Eating olive oil and other monounsaturated fats (as in avocados and nuts) helps prevent memory loss and decline in cognitive function as you age, finds Italian researcher Anthony Capurso, M.D., of the University of Bari. Among a group of 278 elderly Southern Italians, those who ate the most olive oil cut their odds of memory loss by one-third! Most remarkable, olive oil preserved cognitive function in less-educated elderly, who are more prone than highly-educated individuals to memory loss with age. The average amount consumed was high: 3 tablespoons of olive oil daily because Italians use olive oil extensively in cooking. Researchers suggest olive oil, like fish oil, helps maintain the "structural integrity of neuronal membranes," and contains antioxidants that combat brain-cell-destroying free radicals.

OILS WITH THE MOST
BRAIN-BUSTING OMEGA-6S

| Oil | Percentages of | |
---	Omega-6	Omega-3
Safflower, regular	77	
Sunflower, regular	69	
Corn	61	1
Soy	54	7
Walnut	51	5
Sesame	4	1
Peanut	3	3
Canola	22	10
Flax	16	57
Olive	8	1

SOURCE: U.S. Department of Agriculture

Seven Ways to Keep Inflammatory Fats Out of Your Brain

- Don't use corn oil, regular safflower, or regular sunflower seed oils.
- Don't use margarines made from the above oils.
- Don't use salad dressings and or/mayonnaise made with the above oils.
- Don't eat processed foods, such as chips and popcorn, that have been fried, baked, or popped in the above oils.
- Use canola oil (it contains omega-6s, offset with omega-3s for an excellent ratio of 2:1) and olive oil.
- Use flaxseed oil; it has the best ratio of omega-6s to omega-3s. In studies, it relieved manic depression.
- Eat fatty fish (salmon, mackerel, herring, sardines) packed with omega-3s that help neutralize omega-6s.

Amazing New Ways Fish Oil Saves Your Brain

Up from Eden: Why Your Brain Demands
Omega-3 Fat

Since the dawn of mankind, an essential fat, called omega-3, has injected vitality into human brains. It is the stuff that enabled us to finally rise above the other species and create rich civilizations, says Michael Crawford, Ph.D., eminent British authority on brain nutrition at the Institute of Brain Chemistry and Human Nutrition, the University of North London. Dr. Crawford points out that for several million years, evolution of the hominid brain was stuck at a small size of 400–500 grams, a mere pound. The main reason: Early man in landlocked areas of Eurasia lacked the omega-3 fat from seafood needed to spur brain cell growth.

Then over the last million or so years, brain capacity, especially in the cerebral cortex, exploded rapidly in our prehistoric ancestors living in East Africa near large freshwater lakes, says Dr. Crawford. Expanded brain capacity made possible the beginnings of culture—art, music, religion, boat-building, written language, and new social patterns. It's no accident, says Dr. Crawford, that our greatest ancient civilizations arose in areas where humans had access to food from the water—the Nile, Tiber, Euphrates, Ganges, Yangtze (Chang). His contention: Eating seafood with omega-3-type fat was the nutritional stimulus needed to produce huge jumps in brain size and brainpower, tripling brain weight to the current three pounds. With it came a new rush of human achievements.

Today everyone everywhere has access to this precious brain food. But few understand its powers. Thus, we are eating less omega-3 fats and the consequences are grim, according to Dr. Crawford. Brain capacity is no longer increasing, he says. "It's actually going down. I find what's happening now very alarming. The current reduction in omega-3 consumption correlates with an upsurge in brain dysfunction, more mental disease, and lower IQs. Mental defects are on the rise." In short, the evolution of the human brain is in reverse; our brains are now very slowly shrinking, he says. And this trend will continue, he fears, unless we return to the omega-3-rich brain-stimulating diets of our early Paleolithic ancestors.

"The genetic component of intelligence in Britain is declining by about half an IQ point per generation."
—Dr. Richard Lynn, University of Ulster

Failure to eat enough omega-3 fat is scientifically linked to an array of modern mental disorders and problems: depression, poor memory, low intelligence, learning disabilities, dyslexia, attention deficit disorder, schizophrenia, "senility," Alzheimer's disease, degenerative neurological diseases, multiple sclerosis, alcoholism, poor vision, irritability, hostility, inattention, lack of concentration, aggression, violence, suicide.

How Fish Oil Creates Smarter, Happier Brain Cells

How is it possible that the unique fat in fish could have profound effects on the brain? Recent scientific investigations turn up several probable explanations: An abundant supply of fish oil can help defeat free radicals that destroy brain cells, reduce immune responses that trigger cell-damaging inflammation, change the behavior of neurotransmitters, and modify the basic physical structures of brain cells themselves.

Particularly fascinating and important is what happens to brain function when you alter the fat composition of brain cell membranes. Each brain cell, including its long and sinewy branches or dendrites, is covered by a delicate membrane that both keeps out unwanted intruders and controls the cell's internal workings through signaling mechanisms, called receptors, embedded in the membrane. Essentially, the membrane consists of two layers of fatty molecules (phospholipids), and the membrane's flexibility depends on the consistency of its fat. If the fat is hardened like lard, the membrane is stiff and rigid; if the fat is more fluid like fish oil, the membrane is soft and pliable.

Cell membranes must be pliable and in constant flux to perform the communication miracles of the brain, says Dr. Joseph R. Hibbeln, a research psychiatrist at the National Institutes of Health in Bethesda, Maryland. That is especially true, he says, in the synapses of brain cells—the junctions where nerve cells converge to pass their messages. These "synaptic gaps," where signals jump from one cell to another, are the source of the brain's awesome powers. The more of these transmission centers or synapses on brain cells and the smoother the communication between them, the better your brain functions.

Moreover, the number and quality of synaptic connections determine intelligence and optimal brain function even more than the total number of brain cells does. Omega-3 fish oil, more precisely the part called DHA (docosahexaenoic acid), is the building material for synaptic communication centers. You can't create more synapses, dendrites, or receptors that increase your brain's potential without a robust supply of DHA type omega 3-fish oil.

How Fat Manages Messages

Millions of messages pass through the synapses of a cell hourly. To accomplish that, a chemical messenger—a neurotransmitter—is cast adrift into a watery void by one nerve cell to find its way into the receptors of a nearby nerve cell. The event is much like the docking between two spaceships. If the neurotransmitter does not perfectly fit into the receptor or "docking bay" of the waiting neuron, the attempted communication fails. When a transmitter does lock in, it activates the cell to "fire," and release more neurotransmitters to traverse thousands more synapses in a perpetual chain reaction of tiny sparks among billions of brain cells that ultimately form our universe—our thoughts, actions, and mood.

Each neurotransmitter, such as serotonin or dopamine, has a unique shape that must fit into the receptor "docking bay" embedded in the cellular surface membrane. For the perfect fit needed to activate clear transmission, the receptor alters its shape slightly. If the membrane is made of squishy fluid fat, such as fish oil, the receptor can easily change configuration. But if the membrane is made of rigid hard fat, the receptor is immobilized, unable to wiggle or expand to let the neurotransmitter lock in. Then, the communication between cells is not activated, in fact is short-circuited, garbled, muted, or instantly terminated.

Thus, how efficiently neurotransmitters pass from neuron to neuron depends on the fluidity of microscopic fat globules in the synaptic membranes. You can amplify message transmission across synapses a thousandfold by altering fat membrane consistency, says NIH's Dr. Hibbeln. Even if you have an ample supply of chemical neurotransmitters, the message can't get through if the receptors don't function properly. "You can send out all the neurotransmitters you want," says Dr. Hibbeln, "but if only 50 percent of the normally functioning receptors are in a state to activate the messengers, only 50 percent of the message gets through."

In short, a receptor sitting in a cell membrane filled with rigid fat is a dead or mute receptor. It can't sense or transmit much of anything. That is something to remember the next time you set out to solidify your cell membranes by eating butter, french fries, hamburgers, potato chips, and fatty milk shakes, cakes, cookies, and candies.

> **BOTTOM LINE:** *Omega-3s are the most fluid fats for keeping cell-membranes soft and flexible. Animal fats turn membranes crystalline and rigid.*

Additionally, fat's influence on how a brain cell conducts business does not end at the cellular border. Researchers have recently discovered that after a neurotransmitter successfully penetrates the fatty membrane, gaining entry to the heart and soul of the cell, it sets off a cascade of events called a "second messenger system." The neurotransmitter spews off secondary emissaries that reach into the very nucleus of the cell where they turn genes on and off. Further, the genes then feed back chemicals to the outside surface membrane of the cell, creating more reactions. This means that although the receptor is the gatekeeper, plenty happens to neurotransmitters once inside cells that influence mood, behavior, and overall brain functioning. Here again the type of fat in the membrane helps control the generation and recycling of these internal second messengers, turning them up or down, on or off—for good and for ill. Turning up the volume too high on these second messengers can cause static in brain cells, bringing on depression, mania, perhaps even schizophrenia. Fish oil, like certain psychiatric drugs, is thought to suppress an unwanted flood of second messengers bent on havoc.

Fish Secret: Feel-Good Serotonin

An intriguing way fish oil also seems to influence mood and behavior is by boosting brain levels of the feel-good neurotransmitter serotonin. It's well documented that many people with abnormally low brain and blood levels of serotonin are depressed, at high risk of suicide, and criminally "impulsive," for example, are more apt to commit unpremeditated murder, and set fires.

However, if you have high levels of DHA fish oil in your blood, you're apt to have high amounts of serotonin in your brain. In normal people, Dr. Hibbeln has found that the higher the DHA, the higher the serotonin. Thus, he can predict how much serotonin is in your brain by measuring your blood levels of DHA fish oil. Thus, it's logical that you can boost brain serotonin by eating fatty fish that raises DHA blood levels. "And if you have higher serotonin, you would expect less depression, impulsivity, and suicidal behavior," says Dr. Hibbeln.

Precisely how fish oil manages to boost serotonin is not well understood, but scientists speculate it may happen several ways. Changing the fat composition of membranes alters the actions of critical enzymes that, for example, convert tryptophan to serotonin and control its breakdown and reuse or "re-uptake" cycles. There's also recent evidence that eating fish creates more serotonin simply because the body uses DHA fish oil to manufacture more synapses with more nerve endings that in turn produce more serotonin. "It's like building more serotonin factories, instead of just increasing the efficiency of the serotonin you have," explains Dr. Hibbeln.

> **BOTTOM LINE:** *Evidence suggests that fish oil helps regulate serotonin, a neurotransmitter known for its "feel-good" qualities. Depressed, suicidal, impulsive, and violent persons often have low levels of serotonin.*

Another powerful way omega-3 fish oil can guard the brain is by combatting inflammation in cerebral blood vessels and brain cells. Inflammation is increasingly recognized as a villain underlying destruction of brain tissue and function, leading to strokes, even Alzheimer's. Omega-3 restrains production of highly inflammatory hormonelike substances—prostaglandins, leukotrienes, and cytokines— that injure blood vessels and interfere with neurons' message transmission. The more bad omega-6 vegetable fats (corn oil, safflower, sunflower, soybean oil) you eat, the more omega-3s you need to dampen brain-destroying inflammation.

The whole prospect is mind-boggling: The type fat you eat changes the tiny structures of brain cells. This minor change, when multiplied by the billions, alters your brain functioning and consequent behavior. As research psychiatrist Dr. Norman Salem, acting scientific director at the National Institute on Alcohol Abuse and Alcoholism, eloquently puts it: "This may be the only case in modern-day biology where a change in structure at the atomic level can alter the behavior of the whole organism." In short, modifying the chemical composition of tiny fat molecules in your brain cells can quietly, quickly, and profoundly alter your internal self, your identity, who you really are—how you feel, think, and behave.

A Guide to the Mighty Brain Fats

To make your brain work at top form, you need a delicate balance of two essential chemical entities—so-called omega-3-type fish oil and omega-6-type vegetable oils. How much you eat of each dictates the architecture and activity of your brain.

Most important to brain function is omega-3, made up of two specific fatty acids: DHA (docosahexaenoic acid) and EPA (eicosapentaenoic acid).

- DHA—King of the brain fats: Of all brain fats, the DHA part of omega-3 fish oil is the most powerful player in brain chemistry. It constitutes fully one-half of all fat in brain cell membranes. DHA is concentrated where it counts—in the membranes of the synaptic communication centers, in the cerebral cortex (the brain's "thinking center"), in neurons' internal energy factories called mitochondria, and in the photoreceptors of the retina of the eye. DHA is unique in its fluidity, needed to build and preserve pliable brain cell structures that can efficiently conduct the brain's business. DHA also increases supplies of acetylcholine (the memory chemical) in the brains of laboratory animals and reverses their impaired learning performance. The brain grabs most of the DHA you eat to fuel its activities.

  Important: One other thing, adults—not infants—can convert a short-chain fatty acid called alpha-linolenic acid (LNA) into the DHA powerhouse. You get alpha-linolenic acid in green leafy vegetables, flax seed and flax seed oil, canola oil, walnuts, Brazil nuts, seaweed, and algae—not at the top of most Americans' menu. Even so, it's virtually impossible for your body to make enough DHA to meet your brain's demands. You must continually supply your brain cells with already-formed DHA by eating omega-3-rich seafood. Otherwise, your brain falters and malfunctions.

- EPA—Another crucial brain fat: For many years, researchers focused on the EPA fraction of fish oil in regulating blood factors and preventing heart disease. Now scientists know EPA is also vital to the brain. Although normal brain cells contain very little EPA, a lack can bring on mental disorders, and replenishing EPA has improved brain function, especially in schizophrenia. EPA can also be transformed in your body to DHA.

- The two-faced Omega-6s: Omega-6 fatty acids can contribute to brain function, but they are unpredictable and potentially dangerous—often considered bad guys because we eat so much of them that they overwhelm and nullify the crucial brain fats, such as DHA. Eating too much omega-6, for example, can destroy DHA. Still, linoleic acid, the parent or precursor of the omega-6s, can transform itself into more desirable long-chain fats—gamma-linolenic acid (GLA), which then turns into arachidonic acid, another fat required for infant brain development. Arachidonic acid, however, has Jekyll-Hyde characteristics, and in excess can generate chemical reactions that damage cells.

Most important of all: It's not just how much omega-3 fish oil you eat, it's how much you eat compared with how much omega-6 vegetable fats you take in. The ratio is far more critical than the total amount. For example, the Japanese eat as much omega-6 as Americans; but the Japanese also eat thirty times more omega-3. If you examine their tissue, you typically find an excellent ratio of the essential fats.

TEN FISH WITH THE MOST "SMART FATS"

Here's the seafood with the most brain-stimulating DHA. Note: The more fat, the more DHA—high-fat fish is what you want.

Grams of DHA in 3¹/₂ ounces raw or canned

Anchovy	.9
Bluefish	.8
Herring	1.0
Mackerel	1.4
Sablefish	.9
Salmon	.8
Sardines	1.0
Lake trout	.5
Tuna, bluefin	.9
Whitefish	.9

Lower-fat fish, such as cod, catfish, flounder, grouper, haddock, perch, snapper, sole, swordfish, and shellfish contain little omega-3, averaging only .1 to .2 grams of DHA per 100 grams. Source: U.S. Department of Agriculture

Fish eat algae that they convert to DHA; they also eat each other, providing oodles of DHA and EPA and that's why they are so rich in omega-3 brain fats. That's why fish is truly "brain food."

BOTTOM LINE: *You need fish oil to build strong brains and to make them operate at top form for a lifetime. Omega-3 alters brain cell structure and the ability of messages to get through with high-powered transmission.*

HOW THE JAPANESE
BUILD BETTER BRAINS

In Japan, health authorities do not cavalierly sit by and let precious brains go malnourished. In Japan, twenty different foods are fortified with DHA, the fish oil fraction essential for top functioning brains. Such foods include those for infants, such as powdered milk and rice porridge used as a weaning food. (Remember, American infant formula is not spiked with DHA and is considered scandalously inadequate by many scientists.) In Japan, high omega-3 salad dressings (made with perilla oil) are commonly used. Japanese officials also advise pregnant women to eat fish daily to make sure the fetus gets the DHA required for optimal brain development. As fish consumption declines in Japan among young people who are shifting to a Westernized diet, Japanese health officials consider food fortification with DHA fish oil all the more important.

DHA for Test Takers

"Taking DHA supplements before an exam makes sense," says Barbara Levine, Ph.D., chief of nutrition, New York Hospital-Cornell Medical Center. She also favors DHA supplements for pregnant and lactating women, as well as eating fish, because Americans have among the lowest blood levels of DHA in the world. Dr. Levine takes 200 milligrams of DHA daily.

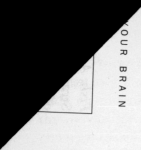

Antidepressant

...seem, eating fish dramatically cuts your ...nto a major depression. It's a truism ...orld, according to research by NIH psy- ...t. Hibbeln. Clearly, he says, depression ...erica in the last half century have steadily increased as fish-eating has declined. The Japanese, the world's biggest fish-eaters (about 140 pounds per year) have the world's rock-bottom rate of major depression, a mere 0.12 percent, according to impeccable scientific data. New Zealanders who eat scant fish (only 25 pounds per person per year) have a 5.8 percent incidence of depression, fifty times more than the Japanese. Americans average about 50 pounds of fish yearly and have a depression rate of 3 percent. Indeed, it is a nearly perfect correlation, Hibbeln finds, between countries with low fish intake and high rates of major depression. In follow-up research, Hibbeln found the same thing true for postpartum depression in women. The condition declines, the more fish a country consumes.

Further, the biological signs of not eating fish show up in the blood of depressed patients. Depressed patients tend to have less omega-3-type fish fat in their blood cells. And the blood level of omega-3 predicts the severity of depression. The lower the omega-3 levels, the more severe the depression. Conversely, the more omega-3 fat depressed patients eat in their normal diet, the less severe their depression.

A recent Australian study of 21 depressed patients confirmed that the most severely depressed had imbalances of fatty acids, mainly rock-bottom levels from fish oil, in their blood and cell membranes. Why? Evidence suggests DHA-type fish oil helps regulate serotonin, a neurotransmitter known for its "feel-good" qualities. Depressed persons often have low levels of serotonin.

THE BRAIN-HEART CONNECTION

It's fascinating to note that those who skimp on fish throughout the world have the greatest incidence of both depression and heart disease. Since it's now known that the fat in fish can protect arteries from clogging and the heart from shutting down, as well as the brain from depression, this may help explain why depression often precedes and predicts heart disease and why the two often strike the same individuals. Hippocrates said it first: "Food that is good for the heart is likely to be good for the brain."

Natural Lithium: A Cure for the Highs and Lows

The big question: If a deficiency of fish oil in neurons helps trigger depression, can it be relieved by taking fish oil? Striking new evidence says it can. In a groundbreaking 1998 study, Dr. Andrew Stoll, a psychopharmacologist and assistant professor of psychiatry at the Harvard Medical School, found that doses of fish oil did indeed relieve bipolar (manic) depression in a group of thirty patients, ages eighteen to sixty-five. Half of the patients, who were all judged "very ill," having had at least four episodes of mania, depression, or both in a year, took about ten grams of fish oil a day (14 very large capsules) made up of a combination of EPA and DHA. The other half took placebo capsules of olive oil. Some patients were also taking conventional medication, including lithium; eight were not.

The results were so startling that Dr. Stoll stopped the study prematurely after only four months instead of the planned nine months. Fully 65 percent of the bipolar patients got better on fish oil compared with only 18 percent on placebo. Moreover, once well, the fish-oil takers stayed well. Only 12 percent on fish oil had a recurrence of depression or mania compared with 52 percent on placebo. Thus, those not getting fish oil were four times more apt to have a manic or depressive episode than those on fish oil. "Surprisingly, the omega-3 patients stayed virtually well," concluded Dr. Stoll.

Some patients were so improved, they lowered their doses of medication or completely dropped it and continued on the "monotherapy" of fish oil alone. Further, the oil often worked "very quickly," says Dr. Stoll, "within a week or two."

Dr. Stoll has high praise for fish oil: "It has a wide spectrum of activity—it appears to be antidepressant, antimanic, and a mood stabilizer. It's extremely safe, well-tolerated, causes no sedation, or other adverse side-effects common in standard drugs." Nor are there interactions with standard treatment drugs, lithium, and valproate, or with other pharmaceuticals with the possible exception of coumadin, an anticoagulant.

Dr. Stoll recommends starting with a dose of five grams per day of fish oil. Capsules, as noted on labels, contain varying doses of DHA and EPA. Generally, it takes seven to eight capsules daily to make five grams, he says. To make the fish oil more palatable, it can be taken with orange juice. Taking most of it at night also cuts down on the fishy aftertaste. At doses of over ten grams daily, fish oil may cause occasional diarrhea or oily stools. The maximum dose used by Dr. Stoll is 15 grams daily.

Flaxseed Oil: The Other Antidepressant?
So encouraged is Dr. Stoll by fish oil therapy for bipolar depression that he continues to give it to patients. However, one day, a patient mistakenly picked up flaxseed oil

instead of fish oil at a health food store. She took it for several weeks and felt so much better that Dr. Stoll now gives flaxseed oil to some patients. Flaxseed oil is a highly concentrated "short-chain" form of omega-3 fat known as linolenic acid. In order for flaxseed oil to possess the chemical aspects and presumed powers of long-chain fish oil, the body must convert flaxseed oil from a short chain to the long-chain fish oil components—DHA and EPA. "I'm not sure why," says Dr. Stoll, "but flaxseed oil also appears to work as an antidepressant and mood stabilizer." One drawback: Some patients on high doses of flaxseed oil have experienced manic episodes.

From two to six tablespoons a day of flax seed oil have relieved depression in some individuals.

How did fish oil alleviate manic depression? Dr. Stoll believes fish oil mimics the activity of the big-gun drugs, lithium and valproate, typical treatments for manic depression. Both drugs work by blocking the recycling of so-called second messengers that can cause havoc inside cells. "We think fish oil works much the same way," he says.

The Case of the Four-Week Depression Cure

When she arrived at the hospital in Scotland, the woman in her mid-forties was experiencing so-called "manic psychosis." Her speech was rapid and disjointed; she was delusional and hearing voices. Her long history of manic depression had been mostly controlled by two standard drugs, lithium and valproate. She confessed to having stopped taking her lithium because it "blunted her creativity," although she was still on valproate. Her psychiatrist obtained permission to try a new treatment: omega-3 fatty acids—fish oil—four grams a day containing two grams daily of the reported active agents, EPA and DHA.

The outcome far exceeded anyone's expectations. In fact,

it was astonishing. In one week, the woman's psychosis was gone. In two weeks her speech started to normalize although she was still very irritable. After three weeks her irritability subsided. After four weeks, she was well enough to be discharged from the hospital. Further, she seemed to have recovered forms of emotional feelings and stability, such as empathy, she had not experienced in a decade. Doctors hope that if she continues to take the fish oil, along with her other medication, she will remain mentally stable. Theoretically, people with manic depression, for unknown reasons, may need more omega-3 fish oils than normal people to keep brain cells functional, says NIH psychiatrist and fish oil authority Joseph Hibbeln.

Feel Hostile? Aggressive? Stressed Out? Try Fish Oil

Under mental stress, you're more apt to become aggressive against others. But it's less likely if your brain is under the influence of fish oil. That's the astonishing finding of a recent study of forty-one Japanese students by Tomohito Hamazaki and colleagues at the Toyama Medical and Pharmaceutical University.

Investigators measured aggression on standard psychological tests in September—just before the end of summer vacation when the students were relaxed and unstressed— and then again on December 4 at an extremely high-stress time when they were taking difficult pathology tests and finishing their graduation thesis. The date was "one of the students' busiest and most frustrating days" of the year, said researchers.

However, in the three months between September and December, all students in the study had been taking special capsules. Half took capsules of fish oil, containing 1.5 to 1.8 grams per day of DHA. The other half got "dummy" capsules of soybean oil. They didn't know which they were getting. (The soybean capsules were doctored to give a slight fishy odor.)

Remarkably, the students on the DHA fish oil sailed through the stress overload without showing a whit of expected extra aggression. But aggression shot up an average 9 percent and as much as 46 percent in students taking the dummy capsules. The conclusion: DHA fish oil kept a lid on the students' aggression at times of mental stress. A follow-up study did not find that fish oil curbed ordinary aggression in students who were not stressed out.

Interestingly, it's possible the extra fish oil had a pharmacological effect and did not fill in a deficiency, for Japanese typically already have high levels of DHA in their blood from eating fish. That means fish oil would be expected to have a much greater impact on lowering aggression in overstressed Americans and other Westerners who are already severely deficient in DHA-type fish oil.

Dr. Hamazaki speculated that keeping the body calm during stress may also help explain how fish oil diminishes heart disease. Stress hormones triggered by anger and hostility can constrict arteries and accelerate formation of blockages, research shows, possibly triggering heart attacks.

Think Faster, Concentrate Better

It was an unexpected and exciting discovery. Dr. Antolin M. Llorente, Ph.D., of Baylor University, set out to do a study of 140 pregnant women to determine if taking fish oil would help prevent postpartum depression, as some evidence suggests. The women were all healthy, well educated, and urban middle class. In the double-blind trial, every day for four months after the baby's birth, half of the women took 200 milligrams of DHA fish oil, and half took a placebo. For various reasons, the study did not pan out in judging the value of DHA for postpartum depression. However, as part of the study, Dr. Llorente measured the change in the fatty acid composition of their blood to make sure DHA levels had risen. On a hunch he also decided to measure the women's mental functioning with a standard test called the Stroop Color Word Test.

Amazingly, he found that taking DHA, according to the test, actually improved the women's mental functioning, notably their concentration and attention. What makes this remarkable, says NIH investigator Dr. Joseph Hibbeln, is that increasing DHA in the blood boosted mental function in women who were in top health and nutritional condition. Does this mean even the most well-nourished Americans are getting less than optimal levels of fish oil for top brain functioning? And that seemingly normal, well-nourished, well-functioning brains can function even better when they get more DHA? Probably. It helps prove the point that in America a normally functioning brain is not an optimally functioning brain. As NIH investigator Dr. Jerry Cott observes, "If a person has so-called 'normal' levels of DHA, you would not expect to get an immediate dramatic benefit from eating fish or taking fish oil."

DHA Speeds Up Brain Waves

Indeed, there's striking new evidence that eating omega-3 fatty acids from fish can speed up brain efficiency in normal persons, as reported by Japanese investigator K. Myanaga at a 1998 international scientific conference in Barcelona, Spain. He studied the impact of fish oil on the speed of a particular brain wave called "p300," closely linked to learning and memory. It is known that the faster the transmission rate of this brain wave, the more efficiently the brain learns and remembers information. For example, the rate of "p300" brain wave declines with age and is much slower in people with dementia.

Dr. Myanaga hooked up electrodes to the heads of twenty-six normal adult volunteers and measured the transmission rate of their p300 brain waves. Then he immediately gave them supplements of DHA or EPA. After two hours, he measured the rate of their brain waves again. Sure enough, he found that the p300 rate was significantly faster in people given DHA, but not EPA. He concluded that "DHA appears to be an exciting drug which can improve brain function . . . in healthy persons."

DHA-Fed Rats Learn Better

In a series of experiments, Japanese researchers studied the effects of fish oil on rats that are prone to high blood pressure and strokes. These rats, compared with normal rats, typically do poorly on certain passive-avoidance learning tasks. But feeding the learning-impaired rats DHA fractions of fish oil virtually reversed their learning deficits. Further, DHA suppressed development of high blood pressure and strokes and extended the animals' lifespans.

Most revealing, when researchers measured neurotransmitters in the brains of DHA-fed rats, they found much higher levels of acetylcholine (the learning and memory chemical) in the hippocampus, indicating DHA revved up formation of this critical neurotransmitter. Moreover, the higher levels of acetylcholine paralleled the degree of improvement in learning, suggesting that DHA mended the dysfunction in brain cells due to acetylcholine deficiency and thereby ameliorated learning failure.

Fish Eaters Stay Smarter Longer

Eating fish may help save your brain as you get older. More than a decade ago, Dutch researchers at the National Institute of Public Health tested a group of elderly men (sixty-four to eighty-four years old) for cognitive function on

HOW MUCH OMEGA-3 DO YOU NEED?

An expert committee recommends as an "adequate intake" of omega-3 fatty acids for adults based on eating 2000 calories a day at least 650 milligrams a day of long-chain omega-3s (DHA and EPA). That's the approximate amount in:

- 1 ounce mackerel*
- 1½ ounces herring
- 1½ ounces canned sardines
- 1¾ ounce fresh salmon*
- 3½ ounces canned albacore white tuna
- 3½ ounces swordfish*
- 7 ounces grouper*
- 12 ounces haddock*

*weight before cooking

several standard tests as part of the Zutphen Elderly Study. Also, their food consumption patterns were recorded. Recently, 390 of the surviving men were reexamined to see whether their mental functions had declined.

A major finding: Men who ate more than 20 grams (¾ ounce) of fish daily were only 40 percent as likely to show an impairment of cognitive function as non-fish-eaters. Further, those who consumed the most omega-6-type vegetable oils were two and a half times more apt to be cognitively impaired. Particularly linked to poor brain functioning were margarine, butter, baking fats, fatty sauces, and cheese. The research team, headed by S. Kalmijn and Dean Kromhout, speculate that the bad omega-6 fats contribute greatly to clogged arteries; thus, the brain impairment probably results from vascular damage to blood vessels in the brain.

Researchers also suggested fish may contain brain-protective antioxidants, such as selenium, in addition to omega-3 fatty acids.

> *"I would recommend DHA for everybody in this country, especially if you're a non-fish-eater. Over the last forty years, dietary levels of DHA have been depleted by about 50 percent."* —David Kyle, Ph.D., Martek Biosciences Corporation. (Kyle, age 45, takes 200 mg of DHA daily.)

The Alzheimer's Connection

Eating fish may also protect you from developing dementia or Alzheimer's disease. Indeed, low levels of DHA-type fish oil predict dementia and Alzheimer's disease in older people, according to a blood analysis of 1188 elderly subjects (average age seventy-five) in the famed Framingham Heart Study. Dr. Ernst Schaefer, and colleagues at Tufts University, found that those diagnosed with Alzheimer's disease were twice as apt to have low DHA blood levels. Further, those with low blood DHA had a 67 percent greater risk of developing Alzheimer's in the next ten years. They also were four times more likely to have lower scores on a specific mental abilities test geared to older people called the Mini Mental State Exam (MMSE). Thus, researchers concluded low blood levels of DHA are a risk factor for low mental performance and the development of Alzheimer's disease and other forms of dementia as you age. One contributing reason: Older people lose the ability to synthesize DHA. This means they must consume DHA directly in fish or fish oil to supply the brain with enough DHA to function normally.

Fish oil is even a treatment for Alzheimer's disease. A

team of Israeli-American researchers have recently shown that the right amount of omega-3 fatty acid in capsules dramatically improved memory, mood, and other symptoms in a surprising *81 percent* of a group of patients with Alzheimer's. Previously the investigators at Bar-Ilan University in Ramat Gan had discovered that rats learned better after taking a ratio of one part omega-3 fatty acid and four parts omega-6 fatty acids. They decided to try the same mixture in a test of one hundred Alzheimer's patients; sixty got the omega-3–omega-6 capsule, while forty others got a placebo.

After only one month, the improvement in those taking the fatty acid capsule was striking. Most of them were more cooperative, better organized, in a better mood, had a better appetite, fewer sleep problems, and hallucinations and were more alert during the day. Most important, short-term memory improved in 74 percent and long-term memory in 58 percent. Researchers credited the better behavior and mood to beneficial changes in the fat composition of the membranes of nerve cells.

Schizophrenics Lack the Right Fats

Nobody really knows the cause of schizophrenia. Many theories focus on a disturbance in neurotransmitter systems. A long-time theory holds that too much activity of the neurotransmitter dopamine disrupts certain neuronal pathways. Newer thought implicates other neurotransmitter systems involving glutamate and serotonin. There's likely to be a genetic component. Lately, a growing number of scientists believe tiny abnormalities in the fat composition of cell membranes disturbs brain functioning to a large degree, resulting in schizophrenic symptoms. Some believe patients with schizophrenia have defective antioxidant defenses, allowing fat in their brain cell membranes to be easily oxidized (turned rancid) by free-radical attacks.

Much evidence shows that brain cell membranes in schizophrenics have an abnormal fat content. The membranes are depleted of both omega-3-type fish fat, notably DHA, and omega-6 linoleic acid as well as arachidonic acid (AA). In one study, leading British researcher Dr. Malcolm Peet, of the department of psychiatry at Northern General Hospital in Sheffield, found that red blood cells of schizophrenics had only half as much DHA and omega-6 fats and one-fourth as much arachidonic acid as normal, healthy individuals. (The amount of DHA and AA in blood cells reflects the amount in brain cells.) Further, schizophrenic patients with the greatest deficiencies of DHA and AA fats tend to have the most advanced symptoms, or so-called "negative" symptoms, including emotional blunting, social withdrawal, poverty of speech and activity, and cognitive deficits, which are most resistant to drug treatment.

Brain images of the prefrontal cortex of schizophrenics show that the fats in cellular membranes are being broken down or destroyed at a rapid rate. Therefore, Dr. Peet theorizes that their neuronal membranes are so distorted that neurotransmitters, including dopamine, and receptors are unable to transmit messages properly. Dr. Peet also thinks schizophrenics are defective in metabolizing arachidonic acid, which is also important in facilitating messages.

Thus, it's not that schizophrenics necessarily have a low intake of omega-3s in their diet. It appears they need more than ordinary humans to try to overcome a metabolic disorder that eats up the essential fatty acids faster. Constantly replenishing the fast-disappearing fatty acids may help the famished brain recover totally or partially.

There's growing evidence that eating extra omega-3 can

relieve symptoms of schizophrenia. For example, in a recent test, Dr. Peet and colleagues had twenty schizophrenic patients take a supplement of ten grams per day of concentrated fish oil (MaxEPA) for six weeks. Unquestionably, cell membrane levels of omega-3 fatty acids shot up, and the higher they went, the more the patients improved, particularly in "negative" symptoms.

So impressive is the evidence that fish oil can help schizophrenics that a new large-scale double-blind multicenter study in the United States is under way, sponsored by the Stanley Foundation, a private research group.

The Incredible Non-Shrinking Brain: A Case History

It's possible that fish oil may stop and even reverse structural disintegration in schizophrenic brains. Scientists know schizophrenic brains look different on PET scans than normal brains. Such images reveal organic brain abnormalities, verifying that the symptoms of schizophrenia are not vague, illusory shadows in the mind, but are engraved into the mass of living brain tissue itself.

Typically the ventricles—normal, fluid-filled spaces—in the brain tend to enlarge in many schizophrenics, especially those in the later stages of the disorder, indicating a loss or shrinkage in brain tissue as the empty space increases. Now what if something could actually halt that shrinkage, as documented by brain images? It would be an astounding event, say experts. But British researcher Basant K. Puri, a specialist in brain imaging and schizophrenia at London's Hammersmith Hospital, has shown that fish oil given to a schizophrenic patient did indeed halt, even slightly reverse, the enlargement of the ventricles common in the progress of the disorder.

In 1996, Dr. Puri suggested that a twenty-eight-year-old with worsening symptoms of schizophrenia of fifteen years' duration (including delusions and hallucination) begin taking 2000 milligrams of EPA fish oil daily. The man was not on antipsychotic medication at the time. Within a month, he felt and looked better. After two months, he exhibited "a dramatic remission, to the point of being normal" in behavior and according to objective tests of symptoms, says Dr. Puri. Over the next six months, his test scores reflected his progressive improvement. He continued to take the omega-3 fish oil and "today is symptom-free," Dr. Puri told an international conference at the National Institutes of Health in September, 1998.

More astounding, Dr. Puri revealed details of PET scan images of the patient's brain before and after he took the omega-3 fish oil. As expected, in 1996 the man's brain showed ventricular enlargement—a shrinking of brain tissue. Only six to eight months after starting to take EPA fatty acids, the loss of brain tissue, as indicated by the worsening expansion of the ventricle holes, "came to an abrupt halt," reports Dr. Puri. In fact, brain pictures taken two years later show that the ventricles actually regressed, so they are smaller now than they were in 1996, and are similar to those in a normal brain. Mind-boggling as it seems, the fish oil appears to have not only stopped but reversed the brain loss, and restored normal brain structure.

As Dr. Puri notes, the astonishing normalization of brain structure and the gradual disappearance of schizophrenic symptoms occurred simultaneously with the consumption of fish oil.

Fish Oil Blunts Brain Damage

If you are a heavy drinker, you may take some comfort in the fact that fish oil may help save your brain from alcohol-induced damage. Dr. Norman Salem, at the National Institutes of Health, explains that excessive alcohol depletes brain levels of omega-3s, DHA in particular, leading to neurological damage and visual impairment. He put experimental animals on high-alcohol, low omega-3 fish oil diets for six months to three years. They suffered severe losses of DHA in brain cells and detrimental changes in brain functioning. Drs. Salem and Hibbeln are planning studies to determine if giving human alcoholics fish oil can mitigate brain damage.

Is Attention Deficit Disorder a Fat Deficiency?

It's a theory that doesn't go away: That certain behavioral problems in children, notably attention-deficient disorder (ADD), also called ADHD when hyperactivity is involved, are related to a deficiency of the right kind of fatty acids in the diet and in brain cells—mainly a lack of omega-3s. The theory goes that such children as well as adults with the disorder may have a genetic glitch that interferes with their ability to metabolize needed brain fats, so they need more of such fats than other brains to function normally.

British researchers Dr. Puri and coresearcher Alexandra J. Richardson, of the University of Oxford, theorize that the activity of a particular enzyme in the brain, delta-6 desaturase, is required to turn on the building blocks or precursors that supply essential fatty acids, including omega-3 and omega-6, to neurons. However, in individuals with ADD, the activity of the needed enzyme is blocked, so that the proper fatty acids are not produced. The result: a kind of famine in the brain, leading to a myriad problems, including learning disabilities, inattention, lack of focus, and hyperactivity.

What blocks the enzyme that turns on production of the brain-essential fats? The two scientists suspect that an inborn weakness in the enzyme's activity makes some youngsters much more genetically vulnerable to ADHD. Psychological stress and a zinc deficiency also block enzyme action, they say. But a major villain that alarms Dr. Puri is overeating bad fats, such as saturated animal fats, hydrogenated fats, and trans fats in margarines and processed foods. All these fats kill the ability of the enzyme to produce vital brain fats. "Whole generations of children live on junk food," laments Dr. Puri, "and it's terrible to think what it's doing to their brains. Fatty junk food not only causes deficiencies, but, worse, it's positively toxic to the brain because it keeps the body from creating essential fatty acids."

Of course, not everyone who eats junk food has overt attention deficient disorder, although Dr. Richardson suspects that high bad-fat diets may be causing unsuspected subtle harm in brain functioning in large parts of the population. Certainly ADD, she says, is caused by several factors, perhaps a fat deficiency as well as genetic predisposition.

Other researchers support the idea of a genetic component to ADD, noting the problem does "run in families." Essentially, they say, the brains of ADD youngsters are running low on essential fatty acids because they have a genetic inability to convert short-chain fatty acids in the diet to long-chain fatty acids that the brain needs to function properly. In short, there seems to be a kind of predisposition to develop the disorder in some youngsters.

At Indiana's Purdue University, Drs. John R. Burgess and Laura Stevens documented that boys ages six to twelve with low blood levels of long-chain omega-3 blood levels were much more apt to have ADD along with other behavioral and learning problems, including impulsivity, anxiety, temper tantrums, and sleep problems.

Lots of Testimonials, Little Proof
The obvious question: Can you overcome attention deficit disorder by flooding the brain with the needed fats? Do

doses of omega-3 and other "essential fatty acids" correct fat deficiencies and brain dysfunction, easing the behavioral problems?

It's unclear. Some experts think it's possible, despite little scientific proof. Two recent double-blind studies, one at Purdue, the other at Baylor University, found no significant improvement in ADD youngsters taking omega-3 fatty acids.

Despite the lack of proof that omega-3 can help rehabilitate ADD brains, countless physicians, parents, and sufferers swear it works. That makes fish oil expert Dr. Joseph Hibbeln at NIH reluctant to write off omega-3 as a potential help for ADD. "Something is happening" he says, "even though we're not sure what. You cannot discount the overwhelming number of anecdotal reports of dramatic improvement. I think the jury is still out."

Dr. Hibbeln, however, suggests another reason fish oil may work for certain children. Some of the behavioral problems attributed to ADD may in fact be manic depression or other psychiatric disorders that may be expressed more strongly later in life. In such cases, he says, fish oil could well help normalize the brain and correct behavioral problems.

BOTTOM LINE: *It's worth trying omega-3 supplements to relieve attention deficient disorder, despite lack of proof. If it doesn't cure the problem, it's still likely to improve brain functioning in general, especially in kids who rarely eat fish. Researchers often give omega-3 supplements along with the drug Ritalin, commonly prescribed for ADD.*

HOW TO SPOT A FATTY ACID DEFICIENCY THAT CAN AFFECT YOUR BRAIN

Primary signs, according to Purdue investigators Drs. Burgess and Stephens: excessive thirst; frequent urination; dry skin; dry, unmanageable, "strawlike" hair; dandruff; small, hard bumps on the arms, thighs, or elbows.

Dyslexia: A Brain Fat Deficiency?

When British nutrition researcher Dr. Jacqueline Stordy, then at the University of Surrey, realized her young son James had a learning disability known as dyslexia, she made him eat fish. "I gave him tuna fish Monday, Tuesday, Wednesday, Thursday," she recalls. "He improved tremendously. He moved from a year behind his classmates to a grade level ahead, and is still doing fine," she reported in September, 1998. The experience launched Dr. Stordy on a scientific mission to save other youngsters from the tragedy of life-long academic and learning failure by documenting that they lack essential brain fats. "If you replenish those essential fatty acids, the brain can resume normal functioning," she says.

Further, Dr. Stordy, along with other researchers, believes that similar learning disabilities, including attention deficit disorder (ADD) and hyperactivity, can be relieved by getting the right fats into the brain.

Dr. Stordy contends that youngsters and adults with dyslexia tend to be deficient in omega-3 fats, notably DHA. The greater the deficiency, the more severe the dyslexia.

Dyslexic Brains Are Different

Brain images by magnetic resonance spectroscopy show that the brains of people with dyslexia do not break down fatty acids and incorporate them into their neuronal membranes the way normal people do. This abnormal metabolism may leave them vulnerable to dyslexia. In short, there appears to be a biological basis for dyslexia. Some brain studies at autopsy have shown widespread microscopic abnormalities in the neuronal organization of dyslexic brains, probably due to abnormal prenatal development. One study by Oxford's Dr. Richardson revealed signs of abnormal metabolism of fatty acids in the brains of nine of twelve adults with dyslexia. Research suggests that dyslexics have trouble synthesizing and getting omega-3 fatty acids into brain cells; thus, they need more of the omega-3 than others.

What is dyslexia? Difficulties in learning to read and write, despite adequate general learning abilities and motivation. It affects about 5 percent of the population, usually males.

Dr. Stordy says that dyslexia and attention deficit disorder can be quite similar and "overlap" or occur in the same individuals about 30 to 40 percent of the time. She says both seem to respond to fish oil supplements, confirming a common cause.

> *"Fish is brain food. It is true in terms of intellect, true in terms of mood and depression, true in terms of concentration and attention. And true for a lifetime—from two years before conception to old age."* —Jacqueline Stordy, Ph.D., British nutritionist and researcher

How to Create a Better Brain for Your Baby

If you are pregnant, you must eat omega-3-type fish oil fats. If you are breast-feeding, you must also eat omega-3 fats. And you must feed your infant omega-3 fats—if you want your child to grow up smart. Neither fetal brains, infant brains, nor childhood brains can reach maximum potential without nourishment from omega-3 fats. In fact, without omega-3, young brains and consequent brainpower may be stunted. The evidence is overwhelming.

> "The mental apparatus of the coming generation is developed in [the womb] and the time to begin supplementation is before conception. A normal brain cannot be made without an adequate supply of omega-3 fatty acids, and there may be no later opportunity to repair the effects of an omega-3 fatty acid deficiency once the nervous system is formed." —Wiliam E. Connor, Oregon Health Sciences Center

Pregnant women who eat fish give birth to more fully developed babies, who are less apt to be born premature or have low birth weight. This means they are born with more mature, highly developed brains.

To get the optimal brain fats into a developing fetus, it's best for a woman to start eating a diet high in fish oil long before she becomes pregnant. It takes months, perhaps years, for the maximum amounts to build up in body tissue to be passed on to a developing fetus. Dr. William Lands, a biochemist at the National Institutes of Health and a leading authority on fish oil, says it may take as long as four years to achieve maximum saturation of omega-3 fat in human tissue.

However, if you are pregnant, it's essential to get plenty of omega-3s. Recent research by William E. Connor, of the

Oregon Health Sciences Center, shows that eating fish, specifically sardines, during pregnancy can dramatically boost levels of all-important DHA in newborn infants. For nine weeks, from the twenty-sixth week to the thirty-fifth week of pregnancy, fifteen pregnant women ate a total of 2.6 grams of omega-3 fatty acids daily from fish and fish oil supplements, including one gram of DHA. An equal number of women ate their regular diets without extra fish oils.

During pregnancy, the amount of DHA in fish-eaters' red blood cells soared 52 percent. Not surprisingly, their newborn infants also possessed much more DHA. Infants born to the fish-eaters had 35 percent more DHA in their red blood cells and 45 percent more DHA in their plasma. Since blood reflects the amount of DHA in body tissue, this means such infants also had more essential brain fats and can be expected to have more highly functional brain cells at birth and in the future.

Note: The fish oil was taken during the latter half of pregnancy, the critical time for maximal development of the fetal brain. Interestingly, the more fish oil a mother ate, the higher both her DHA and that of her newborn. One mother consumed the most—an average of 3.1 grams daily. Her newborn had twice as much blood DHA as the newborn of mothers who consumed the least DHA. (Three and a half ounces of sardines contain about one and a half grams of omega-3s and one gram of DHA.)

Pregnant—and lactating—women should be sure to get at least 300 milligrams per day of DHA, say experts. If you cannot get it by eating fish, you must take supplements.

But it does not stop with birth.

ALARMING FACT: A lack of the right fats can create a deficiency in your baby's brain with irreversible consequences.

A DIET FOR DUMB BABY RATS

There is one way to severely limit the learning ability of young rats: Deprive them of brain-building DHA. That's what Japanese researchers have shown. In experiments, they fed pregnant rats diets adequate in and deficient in omega-3 fatty acids. After the rats were born, they subjected them to learning tests. The two-month-old offspring of rats fed the high fish oil diet did wonderfully well—100 percent learned a task after only three tries. In contrast, the progeny of the rat mothers fed a diet lacking fish oil omega-3s were dreadfully dumb. Only 30 to 40 percent of them could learn the task—even after twenty tries!

Breast-Feeding Makes Smarter Kids

Breast milk, nature's best infant formula, contains omega-3 fatty acids, mainly brain-building DHA, in varying amounts, depending on the mother's diet. And breast-fed babies have more DHA in the cortex of the brain than for-mula-fed infants. That's why scientists believe baby's brains thrive on breast milk. At least eight recent studies show that breast-fed infants have higher developmental scores and higher intelligence scores on standard tests later in life. In one especially convincing study of three hundred children, British researchers at MRC Dunn Nutrition Unit in Cambridge delivered human breast milk to premature infants by tube so as to erase the possibility that sucking at the mother's breast might influence the outcome. Sure enough, infants getting mother's milk early in life scored an average 8.3 points higher on IQ tests at age eight than those fed formula instead of mother's milk. This was after researchers accounted for mothers' education and social class. Researchers concluded that the stuff of mother's milk itself was responsible for boosting IQ scores.

In a similar look at 204 three-year-old children of normal birth weight, psychologists at the University of Houston found that breast-fed kids scored an average 4.6 points higher on intelligence tests (the Stanford-Binet and Peabody Picture Vocabulary Tests) than bottle-fed youngsters.

In another long-term British study, breast-fed infants by age eight had better picture intelligence, and by age fifteen had better scores in mathematics, nonverbal ability, and sentence completion compared with children fed formula as infants.

BRAIN ALERT: The number of mothers nursing their babies has dropped since the peak period of the 1980s. Today only 60 percent are nursing in the hospital and only 30 percent for as long as six months.

Further, a study of one thousand children ages eight to eighteen in New Zealand found that not only breast-feeding, but its duration, increased a child's thinking ability and academic achievement. Infants breast-fed for more than eight months scored better throughout childhood and young adulthood on standardized tests of intelligence, reading comprehension, mathematical ability and scholastic ability, teacher ratings of reading and mathematics, and high-school graduation examinations than did bottle-fed infants.

BRAIN FACT: Mother's milk contains about thirty times more brain-essential DHA (fish oil) than cow's milk.

Of course, even breast milk can be low or deficient in DHA if the mother does not ingest enough DHA in fish or supplements. The content of DHA in breast milk ranges from 0.1 percent in women who skimp on fish to 1.4 percent in women who eat a lot of fish—a 1400 percent difference. Perhaps not surprisingly, DHA in the breast milk of American women is much lower than it was fifty years ago. Among the lowest in DHA in the world, American breast milk contains only one-third the amount of DHA as that of Japanese women. However, women can rapidly boost their breast milk's levels of DHA. It can increase, studies show, as much as 69 percent in lactating women getting DHA supplements for as short a time as six weeks, according to Craig Jensen, M.D., assistant professor of pediatrics at Baylor College of Medicine in Houston, Texas. Adding only 200 milligrams of DHA daily to a woman's diet brings breast milk up to acceptably high levels.

During breast-feeding, women must be sure they eat enough omega-3 brain fats to sustain their infant. How much? At least 300 milligrams of DHA per day, according to a group of international experts who convened at the National Institutes of Health in April, 1999. A daily ounce of a high-DHA fish, such as sardines, would meet the "adequate intake" quota.

Best advice: To be sure you get the needed DHA, nursing mothers should take 200 milligrams of DHA as a supplement, says NIH's Dr. Hibbeln.

Right Formula—More Smarts

If you don't breast-feed, the alternative is infant formula. Unfortunately, it's an unhappy choice. Infant formulas sold in the United States, at this writing, are *not fortified with DHA omega-3 fats*, contrary to recommendations by the World Health Organization that formulas should be similar to breast milk. Many scientific groups, including the British Nutrition Foundation and the WHO/FAO Expert Committee on Fats and Oils in Human Nutrition, recommend that DHA and AA be added to infant formulas. Indeed, such fortified formulas have been available throughout Europe and Asia for several years. You can get them in Mexico. But not in the United States or Canada.

> *"It's a scandal that infant formula is not fortified with omega-3. By failing to give kids omega-3 we are breeding them for mental disease, brain dysfunction, low intelligence, low achievement, and antisocial behavior."* —Dr. Andrew Stoll, Harvard University

> *"Eukanuba [makers of dog food] is putting omega-3 in puppy food. I find it sad we're giving it to our puppies but not to our babies."* —Dr. Barbara Levine, professor of nutrition, Cornell University

> *"There is a virtual consensus of specialists in this field that DHA should be added to infant formula, and that it will make formula more like mother's milk."* —Norman Salem, senior scientist, National Institutes of Health

Formula Stunts Babies' Brains

Much research shows that typical American infant formulas deficient in omega-3 are poor substitutes for breast milk and leave a baby's brain starving for essential fatty acids. Failure to get the proper fats to the newborn brain can result in lower intelligence and compromised vision.

The lack of brain fats is more devastating to premature infants, because their brains are not yet fully developed when they are born. Thus, it's even more critical to add the right fats to formulas for preterm infants. Studies show that such infants given formula with DHA fatty acids process information faster than infants fed standard formula. The DHA-fed babies also had better visual attention at twelve months. Their visual acuity was comparable to that of infants fed breast milk. The same thing is true for term infants; standard formula leaves infants deficient in DHA.

PROOF POSITIVE

Compelling evidence that formulas containing DHA and AA (arachidonic acid) boost infant intelligence comes from a new study by psychologists at the University of Dundee in Scotland. Dr. Peter Willatts and colleagues studied forty-four ten-month-old infants who had been fed two different formulas during the first four months of life. Half received an artificial formula devoid of the right brain fats while the other half took a formula fortified with DHA and AA long-chain fatty acids. The idea was to test problem-solving abilities by videotaping and then assessing how an infant intentionally proceeded through three steps to find a hidden toy.

Unquestionably, infants fed the fatty-acid-fortified formula went about the task with more smarts. In fact, such infants were three times more apt to solve the problem and uncover the hidden toy as infants raised on the deficient formula. This means that the long-chain-fortified formula babies had better memories and attention spans, enabling them to plan and execute their intentions. Better problem-solving at this age means higher IQ scores later in life, say researchers.

The most likely explanation for the infants' higher intelligence and performance: The accumulation of long-chain fatty acids in cell membranes of the central nervous system speeds up information processing. This would boost brain efficiency, making infants quicker to plan and execute a solution before becoming distracted and forgetting the final goal. Further, long-chain fatty acids accelerate the maturation of the structures of prefrontal cortex brain cells—the smart center—needed to pay attention and think.

BOTTOM LINE: *Regardless of the basic mechanism, infants fed brain fats in the first four months of life were more intelligent six months later.*

Infants also need DHA and AA in either breast milk or fortified formula early in life to ensure neurological wiring needed for optimal vision later in life. So say researchers at the Retina Foundation of the Southwest and the University of Texas Southwestern Medical Center in Dallas. In one test at age three, 93 percent of the breast-fed group had a perfect score in visual recognition compared with only 61 percent in the cow-milk-based formula-fed group. Further, babies fed DHA-fortified formula for the first seventeen weeks of life had better visual acuity by age one than did infants getting standard formula. DHA-fed infants saw an equivalent of one line better on a typical eye chart!

This suggests, says author Dennis R. Hoffman, that DHA alone or with AA given at a critical early period of development creates long-term changes in the underlying neural structure needed for "optimal development of the human brain and eye."

ALARMING FACT: More than 70 percent of the nation's four million newborns every year exist mainly on infant formula by age three months.

How to Create Brain-Building Formula

If you are using standard formula, you must get brain-building DHA into your infant's diet. Probably the easiest way is to buy DHA capsules at health food stores. Some are derived from fish oil and some from algae. One, called Neuromins™ and made by Martek Biosciences Corporation, comes in soft gel capsules of 100-milligram or 200-milligram doses; the latter is made especially for pregnant and lactating women and has been tested in clinical studies. The DHA is extracted directly from microalgae, which is the fish's dietary source of DHA. Thus, it is a vegetarian product for those who do not want to consume fish or fish products. Pregnant or lactating women can take the capsules.

You can also pierce the capsule and add it to the baby formula. How much? The World Health Organization recommends that infants get 20 milligrams of DHA for every 2.2 pounds of body weight. Thus, a single 100-milligram capsule every other day would suffice for a newborn weighing from six to eight pounds. After a baby weighs about twenty pounds, you can add a 100-milligram DHA capsule every day, say experts.

Thus, you can easily elevate an infant's intake of DHA to levels found in formulas and breast milk, shown to create smarter and better brains.

BOTTOM LINE: *All in all, fish oil is essential at any age for optimal brain functioning. Eat fish or take fish oil supplements, readily available at health food stores and pharmacies. Taking 300 milligrams of EPA and/or DHA omega-3 fatty acids provides as much fish oil as eating a serving of a medium fatty fish.*

The Two Faces of Sugar: Brain Booster and Brain Buster

It may surprise you to learn that your brain is a glutton for the sweet stuff in your blood. Your nerve cells depend on a normal range of blood sugar—not too much, not too little—to function optimally. Indeed, nothing is more critical to your brain than the type of sugar, called glucose, that circulates in your blood and cells, and is largely determined by what you eat. Nerve cells can't survive and thrive without blood glucose, also known simply as "blood sugar." It is nature's original "smart drug" and mood elevator. It can perk up your memory, concentration, and learning abilities. It can help take away the blues and dampen your irritability. Deficiencies of blood glucose can cause the brain to slow down and malfunction. Yet high levels of blood sugar can be extremely detrimental. It can impair brain performance and memory. It can disturb the functioning of susceptible young brains and mangle brain cell architecture, accelerating mental decline as you age.

BOTTOM LINE: *A major secret of superior brain functioning is to eat in ways that give your brain cells steady access to desirable levels of blood sugar.*

A GUIDE TO SUGAR LINGO

The word sugar can be confusing because its meaning is so broad and encompasses both sugar in the diet and in the blood. The sugar you eat is technically a carbohydrate. There are two types of carbohydrates: simple sugars, including sucrose, or table sugar: and complex carbs known as starches, such as potatoes, cereals, fruits, and other vegetables.

Sucrose is refined table sugar.

Fructose is sugar in fruits.

Glucose is sugar in the blood. The main point: All sugars and starches and some fats and proteins, when digested and metabolized, end up as glucose in the bloodstream. Glucose is the energy your body and brain run on. (Concentrated liquid or powdered glucose is also sold in health stores and pharmacies, and used in experimental studies.)

The Brain's High-Octane Fuel

Sugar in the form of glucose is so incredibly important because it powers the brain. Indeed, glucose is the brain's exclusive source of fuel. Other cells can convert fat and protein into glucose in a pinch, but not neurons. Without its glucose fix, the brain fails. Amazingly, although the brain is only about 2 percent of body weight, it can consume 20 to 30 percent of the body's entire energy. Further, the brain stores so little glucose or energy that, if not replenished, it would be all used up within ten minutes!

At any instant, your brain cells are sponging up glucose from your cerebral blood vessels and transporting it to the thousands of tiny energy factories, called mitochondria, within each neuron. There the glucose is processed and burned as fuel to carry out the important business of the brain. If brain cells can't find enough or can't properly handle the requisite glucose, their furnaces burn less intensely, creating an energy crisis. On a wide scale the ultimate result could be a disturbance in memory or mood, or other hitches in brain function. A smoothly functioning brain needs just the right amount of glucose. Small wonder that much new research on brain function focuses on getting proper amounts of glucose to brain cells. Glucose problems can adversely affect memory, attention span, concentration, excitability, mood, and promote dementia and Alzheimer's disease.

How does crucial glucose get in the blood? Mostly from eating sweets and starches, called carbohydrates. A bite of sugar, or starchy potato, bread, or pasta is broken down into glucose molecules in your small intestine, which are then transferred to your blood and brain. All of your cells survive by burning glucose, but the brain is most dependent of all. As Dr. Jennie Brand-Miller, carbohydrate expert and associate professor of nutrition at the University of Sydney in Australia, says, "The body maintains a certain level of glucose in the blood to serve the brain and central nervous system."

This peculiar sugar, glucose, is our lifeline, just as oxygen is. And, like oxygen, glucose has built-in hazards. It can mutilate and destroy cells. As famed biochemist Dr. Lester Packer at the University of California, Berkeley, says, "We can't live without oxygen, or glucose, but both can also be extremely toxic." Because of nature's plan fashioned millions of years ago, he says, we live our entire lives at the mercy of sugar and oxygen. How well we understand and manage those two critical elements greatly influences the functioning of our cells, including our nerve cells, and our susceptibility to the ravages of aging and disease that can steal our brains.

Three Brain Sugar Rules

Here are three essential things you need to know about blood sugar (glucose) and your brain:

1. For optimal brain function, try to maintain "normal" levels of glucose in your blood; extra high or low levels compromise mental function.
2. Fluctuations in blood glucose help regulate cognition and mood—how you think and feel. The amount of glucose in your blood alters memory, learning capacity, and mood. It also influences your vulnerability to diabetes, arterial damage, strokes, dementia, and possibly Alzheimer's disease.
3. You can greatly influence blood glucose fluctuations by what you eat. Carbohydrates—sweets and starches— by far have the most profound direct impact in creating the glucose that powers your brain.

> **BOTTOM LINE:** *Your blood sugar rises and falls, according to the types and amounts of carbohydrates— sweets and starches— you eat. Carbohydrates are converted in the body to glucose which cells, including neurons, use for fuel. Knowing how to manipulate sugar in your blood gives you enormous power over your brain's intellectual and emotional well-being.*

Blood Sugar: A Key to Memory

If your circulating blood sugar levels are abnormally low or high, your memory and learning ability can suffer, according to extensive evidence. Leading pioneers in this field are the husband-wife team of Paul Gold, Ph.D., and

Donna Korol, Ph.D., previously at the University of Virginia and now at Binghamton (New York) University. In a series of experiments with animals and humans, they have demonstrated that blood sugar levels are critical to memory—the ability to store new information and recall it later—at all ages, particularly among older people. "There is a U curve," says Dr. Gold. Too little blood sugar hinders memory; so does too much. How rises in blood sugar from eating carbohydrates affect your brain, he says, depends on several factors, such as current glucose blood level, stress levels (stress hormones raise blood glucose levels), and individual tolerance to glucose. For example, stress tends to ratchet up glucose levels. Thus, eating lots of carbohydrates at a time of high stress, as before taking an exam, could send blood glucose soaring higher than at times when you are not under stress, says Dr. Gold.

One of Dr. Gold's key discoveries: When blood sugar goes up moderately, but not excessively, memory and learning generally improve. Why is not entirely clear, but Dr. Gold's research suggests that elevated blood sugar signals release of the neurotransmitter acetylcholine, well known to help regulate memory formation and learning. Injecting rats with glucose triggers an increase in acetylcholine. Interestingly, however, the animals' brains release extra acetylcholine only when they are stimulated, in the midst of learning new information, but not when they are sitting quietly in their cages. The same thing apparently happens in college students, Dr. Gold observes. Increased blood sugar boosted mental performance only on tests that were difficult and challenging, not on those that were easy. The implication: Glucose was burned up and needed to be replaced only when the brain was working hard. *In short, the harder you use your brain, the more important it is to have adequate blood and brain glucose.*

RULE NUMBER ONE: When your mind is most active, striving hardest to solve a problem or learn something new, your brain burns more glucose. Thus, you must replenish the glucose reserves in your brain to go on learning at an optimal level. If blood glucose reserves are not available, memory and learning decline, according to studies.

A Memory Boost for Aging Brains

Every brain needs glucose, but aging brains may need more. One reason: As you age, your ability to metabolize glucose, especially in the brain, declines. In remarkable experiments, Drs. Gold and Korol have reversed age-related memory impairments in old rats by administering either adrenaline or straight glucose guaranteed to raise blood sugar. So dramatic is the memory restoration that both middle-aged and old rats injected with adrenaline or glucose have memory scores similar to those of young rats. In short, the memory capacity of old rats is almost completely rejuvenated by raising blood sugar levels. Thus, some memory loss due to aging may at least be partially remedied by simply getting a little extra glucose in your blood and brain!

Indeed, Dr. Gold and colleagues showed that certain aspects of memory improved in healthy older people ages fifty-eight to seventy-seven after they drank a large glass of lemonade spiked with 50 grams of carbohydrate found in a concentrated form of pharmaceutical glucose, in comparison with drinking lemonade sweetened with saccharin. After taking glucose, subjects scored nearly 40 percent better on overall memory based on the Wechsler Memory Scale than after taking saccharin. Boosting blood sugar appears to improve "storage" of information and ability to retrieve or recall it later, researchers said. However, there was no improvement in short-term memory, attention, or overall intelligence quotients. In other tests, older people getting glucose did about 40 to 50 percent better on tests of creativity and flexible thinking.

More Glucose vs. Alzheimer's?

Boosting blood sugar levels may also improve memory in Alzheimer's patients. There is evidence glucose's ability to cross the blood-brain barrier and the rate of glucose metabolism are reduced in Alzheimer's patients, suggesting that an abnormality in breakdown of glucose is a contributor to failing cognitive function in Alzheimer's. Dr. Carol Manning, at the University of Virginia, has given drinks sweetened with glucose to Alzheimer's patients with great success. Their ability to recall a prose passage read to them improved by 100 percent in such individuals, equaling benefits induced by powerful pharmaceutical drugs. "The improvement we see with glucose is at least as great as the improvement we see with tacrine or Aricept [approved prescription drugs for Alzheimer's]," Dr. Manning says.

It makes sense, she says, for those with Alzheimer's to eat plenty of carbohydrates to keep blood sugar levels up. There are anecdotal reports of Alzheimer's patients whose memories dramatically improved when given a diet high in carbohydrates, such as pasta, bread, cereal, even sugar, instead of a carbo-restricted diet. In such cases, the benefits appear to outweigh the ordinary risks of high circulating levels of blood sugar.

Why You Can't Learn on an Empty Stomach—Or How Breakfast Makes You Smarter

When you don't eat, your blood sugar levels drop. And that's apt to mean your brain is short on fuel and can't function as efficiently. Thus, it's logical that trying to learn something on an empty stomach is more vulnerable to failure.

When neural activity is stimulated, your brain gobbles up glucose from your blood, so you need to replace it by eating something. That's one reason experts say that eating breakfast is an excellent way to jump-start your brain, and that's especially true for schoolchildren and adolescents. Compelling evidence shows that breakfast can boost brain functioning—learning, memory, academic performance— and general emotional and psychological well-being. The rationale: Breaking an overnight fast by eating breakfast raises supplies of glucose for the brain. Also, regularly eating breakfast over the long term may eliminate nutrient deficiencies known to subvert brain functioning.

> **BRAIN ALERT:** Fewer adolescents are eating breakfast. Between 1965 and 1991, the percentage of fifteen- to eighteen-year-olds eating breakfast dropped from 90 percent to 75 percent among boys and from 84 percent to 65 percent among girls.

Impressive new research by J. Michael Murphy, of the Department of Psychiatry at Harvard Medical School, documents that a school breakfast improves academic performance, psychological well-being, and behavior. He studied hundreds of youngsters in inner-city elementary public schools in Baltimore and Philadelphia. When compared with kids who rarely ate breakfast, those who often ate breakfast (consisting of virtually any type food) had 40 percent higher math grades and were less apt to be absent or tardy from school. A lack of breakfast took a heavy toll emotionally. Non-breakfast-eaters were twice as apt to be depressed and four times as apt to have anxiety. They were also 30 percent more likely to be hyperactive and to have a variety of psychosocial problems compared with consistent breakfast eaters.

Moreover, Dr. Murphy's investigations showed that kids who went from rarely eating to often eating breakfast had big upswings in academic performance. Such youngsters also became significantly less depressed, anxious, and hyperactive.

"When kids who rarely ate breakfast started eating breakfast consistently, their math grades on average soared a whole letter—from a C to B." —J. Michael Murphy, Harvard Medical School

Although malnourished kids suffer most from a lack of breakfast, even well-nourished brains function subnormally when kids skip breakfast. Research at the University of Texas in Houston found that well-nourished nine- to eleven-year-old kids who ate breakfast did better on certain learning tasks than non-breakfast-eaters. This was true of youngsters regardless of IQ, although breakfast boosted learning most in those with lower IQs.

BOTTOM LINE: *Be sure your child eats breakfast every day, but especially on days he or she is taking a test at school. It could mean a higher grade. Your brain burns glucose when you think; if you run low, your mind slows down.*

Tests by leading British psychologist-researcher Dr. David Benton, at the University of Wales-Swansea, confirm that breakfast's boost in blood glucose stimulates learning and memory in adults, too. In one study thirty-three university students either ate no breakfast or drank a breakfast beverage containing 18 grams of protein, 38 grams of carbohydrate, and 12 grams of fat. They then took standardized memory tests. Their blood glucose levels were measured before breakfast and two hours later, after the memory tests. The breakfast eaters had higher blood glucose and faster recall. Higher glucose also predicted more accuracy on the tests, indicating better memory performance.

Dr. Benton has found the same in repeated studies—that eating breakfast improves memory and retention of new information, but does not affect measures of basic intelligence.

As for the best type of breakfast foods, Dr. Benton favors carbohydrates, such as breads, milk, and cereal, but "eating anything in the morning," he says, is "better than eating nothing."

Sugar Excess: An Alarming Epidemic

Undeniably, you need sufficient blood sugar to power your brain. And quick jumps in blood sugar can be beneficial when you are taxing your brain to learn something new or when an aging or demented brain needs extra stimulation. But the truth is millions of American brains are threatened by the opposite hazard: chronically *high* circulating levels of blood sugar and its companion, the hormone insulin. Such high levels of glucose and insulin day after day can result in degradation of memory and mental functioning, partly because of so-called "insulin resistance" or "prediabetes." If you are genetically susceptible, especially if you are overweight, such insulin resistance may also lead to Type 2 diabetes with increasing likelihood of blood sugar control, heart disease, and neurological complications, even Alzheimer's disease.

How You Make Blood Sugar

Here's what happens: When you eat carbohydrate—plain sugar or starch, such as pasta, potato, bread, beans—it is digested and converted mainly into the single sugar molecule, glucose, that is absorbed into the bloodstream. This infusion of glucose signals the pancreas to make more insulin, the hormone needed to usher glucose into the cells where it can be burned as fuel. Insulin's job is to efficiently process the glucose, getting blood sugar levels back to normal.

It usually goes smoothly if blood sugar rises are gradual. But if blood sugar surges too high, too fast, from eating lots of quickly digested carbohydrates, the pancreas must churn out more insulin in attempts to control glucose. If that happens over and over, year after year, the pancreas can become exhausted, eventually putting out insulin that is too weak and insufficient to control blood sugar. The cells then become insensitive or "resistant" to the insulin. The pancreas frantically spews out more insulin to try to clear blood sugar. The potential catastrophic result is a condition called "insulin resistance"—the inability to fully utilize insulin—that can lead to Type 2 diabetes or independently to vascular problems, such as high blood pressure and thickened carotid arteries, affecting the brain.

Insulin resistance is a hallmark of diabetes. Additionally, millions of Americans—an estimated 25 percent of adults—not known to have diabetes are insulin resistant. The condition is a rapidly growing epidemic, tied to high-fat, high-processed-foods diets, with severe consequences for the brain.

> **BOTTOM LINE:** *High levels of blood sugar or glucose create high blood levels of insulin. These twin devils can be hazardous to your brain, blood vessels, and the rest of your body.*

HOW HIGH BLOOD SUGAR AND INSULIN HARM YOUR BRAIN

- High insulin levels are a prelude to high blood pressure, a prime risk factor for intellectual decline in later life.
- High blood sugar and high insulin tend to make arteries more stiff and less elastic, restricting blood flow to the brain.
- High blood sugar and high insulin stimulate a thickening of the walls of the carotid arteries. Such carotid thickening is a major factor linked to a loss of cognitive function with age.
- Insulin resistance is tied to a sensitivity to sodium that tends to raise brain-damaging blood pressure.

The Mental Ravages of High Blood Sugar

There's extensive and growing evidence that your brain rebels against persistent high blood sugar. Undeniably, abnormalities in blood sugar and insulin cause disturbances in memory and brain function. It happens in youngsters and adults, in those with active diabetes and in countless millions who don't even know they have hazardously high blood sugar. The mental toll is most apparent in older people when years of cumulative damage begin to show up as severe loss of memory and intellectual functioning. The clear message: Controlling high blood sugar, and insulin, should be a high brain-saving priority at all ages.

Here's some of the compelling evidence:

Abnormally high blood sugar in diabetic children can cause a significant drop in IQ scores.

Older people with "persistent impaired glucose toler-ance," probably due to high insulin levels, score lower on tests of overall mental function and long-term memory. Older diabetics are three times more apt to show signs of cognitive decline in standard mental testing.

Striking evidence of the dangers of chronic high blood sugar to intellectual functioning comes from the so-called Zutphen Elderly Study by Dutch investigators. In the study, men between ages sixty-nine and eighty-nine were given oral glucose tolerance tests and a standard measure of cog-nitive function called the Mini-Mental State Examination. The results: The number of errors on the mental function test climbed along with levels of fasting blood sugar.

Specifically, known diabetics (with the highest blood sugar levels) made 23 percent more errors on the test, newly diagnosed diabetics, 16 percent more errors, and those with impaired glucose tolerance (prediabetes) made 18 percent more errors than those with normal blood sugar tolerance. Further, *nondiabetics* with the highest blood insulin levels made 25 percent more mistakes on the mental test than those with the lowest insulin blood levels. Nondiabetic sub-jects with impaired glucose tolerance and abnormally high insulin had impaired cognitive function as measured by the routine mental test.

One theory: High insulin might be detrimental to "synaptic activity" in the brain, interfering with message transmission between brain cells, concluded researchers.

High blood sugar predicts strokes. Diabetics have three times the risk of stroke as nondiabetics. Even nondiabet-ics with nonfasting high blood sugar (over 225 mg/dL) have double the odds of "blood clot" stroke than men with low to normal blood sugar, (under 151 mg/dL), according to a recent twenty-two-year study of about 7500 Japanese-American men. High blood sugar did not raise the chances

DIABETES OF THE BRAIN?

It's a new and controversial idea: that insulin affects memory, learning, and general brain function far more deeply than previously thought. Some researchers even contend that neurons, just like other cells, need insulin to process glucose—an idea that flies in the face of long-time conventional belief. Such scientists suggest that insufficient or "low voltage" insulin could starve neurons of glucose, leading to a partial power outage or "brownout" of the brain, resulting in weakened message transmission, a slump in learning, and memory failure of the type seen in age-related impairment and Alzheimer's disease. In a word, memory disturbances due to ineffectual insulin inside brain cells might be a kind of "diabetes" or prediabetes of the brain.

That's what neuroscientist Siegfried Hoyer at the University of Heidelberg in Germany theorizes. He finds that rats with brains made resistant or insensitive to insulin quickly develop memory loss, which progresses to an Alzheimer's-like state. He, as well as neuroscientist Suzanne Craft at the University of Washington, have found insulin disturbances in the brains of Alzheimer's patients. "We believe that some cases of Alzheimer's disease are like diabetes mellitus," says Dr. Hoyer.

of a bleeding or hemorraghic stroke. Further, high blood sugar was tied to more strokes regardless of whether the men had high blood pressure.

Why is unclear. But autopsies show that diabetics have

more severe atherosclerosis in the small blood vessels of the brain as well as in the carotid (neck) arteries that feed the brain.

High blood sugar and insulin encourage age-related dementia (general intellectual decline) and Alzheimer's disease. A recent study at the Mayo Clinic found that Type 2 (adult onset) diabetics were 66 percent more apt to develop all types of dementia, and male diabetics had more than twice the risk of developing Alzheimer's disease. Diabetes tripled the odds of dementia and Alzheimer's in a recent large-scale study at the University of California at Davis.

Main message: A jump in blood sugar levels is okay sometimes (it's normal after eating) and can benefit learning and memory on a short-term basis. Chronic high levels of blood sugar and insulin over long periods of time are dangerous and can be detrimental to optimal brain function.

How to Save Your Brain from High Blood Sugar

What can you do to avoid this brain menace? What makes blood sugar and insulin soar and stay at abnormally dangerous levels? Obviously, genetic makeup influences blood sugar; some people are blessed at birth with good blood sugar control. Others are more genetically vulnerable to developing insulin resistance and diabetes. But genes are far from destiny. Lifestyle, including the foods you eat, can dramatically influence blood sugar and insulin levels and override a predisposition to such conditions. Indeed, evidence shows that the rise in insulin resistance and diabetes is closely tied to diet. Restricting saturated animal fat can go a long way to avoiding and correcting insulin resistance and diabetes. Also critical are the carbohydrates—sweets and starches—you eat, for carbohydrates, especially of the "wrong" type, can spike blood sugar and insulin, often leading to persistent high blood sugar, insulin resistance and diabetes, and possibly compromised mental function.

Brain Perils of Your Diet

Our modern diet is a minefield of hazards to blood sugar normalcy, and quite out of sync with the diet of our ancient ancestors. The prehuman evolutionary diet that formed our brains, mandating high requirements for glucose, was rich in carbohydrates—just as high as ours—about 65 percent of calories. The difference is the type of carbohydrates. The early carbs came from fruits, vegetables, and beans, as well as honey. Ours come from refined sugar and finely processed flour made into blood-glucose-spiking cereals, bread, and other baked goods. Although grains and dairy foods are "new" in evolutionary terms, even they, ten thousand years ago, were quite different in their impact on blood sugar. They were mostly whole grains and yogurt; consequently they produced gradual blood sugar rises that were compatible with good brain function. Today's staples, such as bread, are made from fine-particle flours that fly through our digestive system, spiking our blood sugar.

> "With the advent of high speed roller mills in the nineteenth century, it was possible to produce white flour so fine that it resembled talcum powder in appearance and texture. . . . As a consequence . . . the blood sugar rise after a meal was higher and more prolonged, stimulating the pancreas to produce more insulin. . . . Thus, one of the most important ways in which our diet differs from that of our ancestors is the speed of carbohydrate digestion and the resulting effect on blood sugar and insulin levels." —Dr. Jennie Brand-Miller, University of Sydney in Australia, *The Glucose Revolution*

Unquestionably, carbohydrates, as well as animal fats, can play havoc with blood sugar and insulin, and thus with memory and other mental functions. But this does not mean you must avoid carbohydrates. Because of the newly discovered hazards of carbohydrates in promoting high circulating levels of blood sugar and insulin, as well as obesity, a flurry of popular advice warns against the intake of carbohydrates. This erroneously assumes carbohydrates of all types are hazardous. The confusion comes from a misperception that carbohydrates are equally treacherous in their ability to endanger the brain by dysregulating blood sugar and insulin. That is far from true. Certain carbohydrates nourish your brain without upsetting blood sugar and insulin. The trick is to know which carbohydrates are good for your blood sugar and brain, and which are not.

Your Brain Likes Some Carbs

One of the great contributions to understanding the impact of food on blood sugar and insulin levels is the recent discovery that carbohydrates—sweets and starches—have widely varying and surprisingly unpredictable effects on blood sugar. This is causing a revolution in the way we judge carbohydrates and their potential influence on health in general and mental health in particular.

For the most part, your brain needs steady supplies of glucose supplied by foods that slowly raise blood sugar levels. However, sometimes your brain needs a jolt of glucose to arouse it to its greatest heights. It's interesting that our evolutionary diet was not devoid of such quick sugar boosts. For example, dates, one of our oldest foods—once ironically recommended for diabetics—send blood sugar soaring far more than eating plain refined sugar, candy, or practically any other food.

Best advice: You can and should eat carbohydrates compatible with the type diet your brain best thrives on. It's a matter of knowing which foods those are.

Fast Carbs and Slow Carbs

What is the right stuff to keep your blood sugar optimal and your brain functioning at peak power? Which carbohydrates best sustain blood sugar reservoirs needed by the brain for energy? The answer is of major relevance for brain function, considering the brain is totally dependent on the status of glucose in your blood.

Essentially, you can judge carbohydrates by whether they cause rapid, steep increases in blood sugar or slow, gradual rises, or something in between. Until recently, sugar was deemed the worst villain. For years, scientific dogma held that eating plain sugar zipped right through the digestive tract, causing the most rapid and highest elevations of blood glucose. Conversely, starches, like bread and potatoes, were thought to dawdle in the intestinal tract, leisurely raising blood sugar. That's why sugar was considered anathema for diabetics, but starches okay. It was a seismic scientific shock to learn this long-time belief was a monumental myth.

> *"Eating white potatoes or white bread is just like eating candy, as far as your body knows."* —Walter Willett, chairman of nutrition, Harvard School of Public Health

No question, carbohydrates differ in their powers to raise blood sugar. But it's far more complicated than the notion that simple sugars are "fast" and starches are "slow." New research, beginning in the 1980s, has created a radical new view of how carbohydrates regulate blood sugar. The new scientific truth: *Each food has its own distinctive abilities to raise blood sugar.* And scientists can accurately predict the sugar-raising properties of a food *only by testing it.* They are often quite surprised to find that a fruit, such as dates, causes blood sugar to spike rapidly, while a similar food—dried apricots—does not.

By feeding numerous people carbohydrates and meticulously measuring their blood sugar increases, pioneering researchers have identified each food's unique glucose-boosting potential. Among the startling revelations: White potatoes raise blood glucose faster than plain sugar does; white bread, more quickly than ice cream. This has turned conventional scientific wisdom on its head, forcing a complete re-examination of which foods over the long run are best for the brain, arteries, and general health.

Important new stuff: Technically, carbohydrates that quickly raise blood sugar are called "high glycemic index" or high GI foods—glycemic being another term for sugar. High GI foods can produce spikes and valleys in blood sugar, sometimes creating a feast or famine for the brain. In contrast, carbohydrates that gradually raise glucose are "low glycemic index" or low GI foods. Generally, eating low GI foods discourages sharp peaks and valleys in blood sugar, creating more mental equanimity. Such "slow" carbs also help ward off and reverse insulin resistance with its hazard of memory impairment.

For the first time in human history, because of modern food processing, our diet is centered on huge quantities of high glycemic carbohydrates, refined sugars and starches, that require the pancreatic production of large amounts of insulin day after day for a lifetime. Small wonder, many bodies are not genetically able to meet the demands and develop insulin resistance and Type 2 diabetes. Such disturbances in blood sugar and insulin levels are hazardous to your body and your brain.

The Hazards of "Fast" Carbohydrates

Harvard researchers have found that a diet rich in quickly digested high glycemic index carbohydrates, that swiftly raise blood sugar, doubles or triples your odds of developing diabetes, insulin resistance, and heart disease.

Eating high glycemic index foods frustrates your ability to lose weight, promoting obesity, and Type 2 diabetes. Low GI foods suppress appetite and stimulate the burning of body fat, say Australian researchers. Several weight-loss diets are based on eating low GI foods.

A high glycemic index diet depresses good-type HDL cholesterol, according to a British study of 1400 middle-aged adults. The best dietary way to raise HDLs, they found, was to eat a low glycemic index diet. Possible explanation: A low glycemic diet increases sensitivity to insulin which raises HDLs.

High glycemic index foods lead to "insulin resistance," or "prediabetes" in which insulin becomes ineffective, promoting high blood pressure, clogged arteries, heart attacks, strokes, possibly even Alzheimer's disease, according to research. *Eating a low GI diet for only a few weeks has reversed "insulin resistance"* in both heart bypass patients and young women.

Persistent high blood sugar from eating a high glycemic index diet can also threaten the brain directly by inflicting a form of age-related damage known as "glycation."

The solution to this modern dilemma is to eat carbohydrates that best nourish the brain by keeping blood sugar and insulin levels essentially "normal" and that are consistent with the long-ago diets that formed our brains. That means basing your diet on carbohydrates with a low glycemic index rather than a high glycemic index—foods that cause slow rises rather that rapid spurts in blood sugar and insulin. To do that, you must have accurate information on the glycemic indexes of common foods.

> **BOTTOM LINE:** *It's important to know which carbohydrates spike blood sugar so you can maintain optimal blood glucose levels required to fuel your brain and to stave off potential brain damage.*

The Incredible Carrot Myth and Other Facts

Unhappily, some of the information on the glycemic index values of foods in popular distribution is wildly wrong. Some of the first analyses done in the early 1980s are still being quoted as gospel, even though they are out of date, erroneous, and have been replaced in the scientific arena with findings from newer analyses. A case in point: the carrot.

Because of the tenacity of misinformation, millions of Americans on a supposedly low glycemic index diet (some diabetic, some trying to lose weight, suppress hunger, or gain energy per *The Zone*) are told to shun carrots like the plague; supposedly, carrots send blood sugar levels soaring. Not so. The truth is carrots are actually a low glycemic index food, according to the most recent authoritative tests published in 1999 by the world's leading experts in Australia and Canada. The fact is carrots contain so few carbohydrates (only 5 to 7 percent or a mere 3 grams in half a cup) that to spike blood sugar you would have to eat at least one and a half pounds or five cups at one sitting.

BOTTOM LINE: *Raw, cooked, or canned, carrots are good for your blood sugar and your brain. They do not cause blood sugar surges! Widespread reports that carrots are detrimental to the blood sugar of diabetics, people trying to lose weight, or anyone, for that matter, are "simply wrong," says world authority Dr. Jennie Brand-Miller, at the University of Sydney in Australia, who continually conducts analyses of the glycemic index of foods.*

The Real Guide to Brain-Boosting Carbs

Here is the latest accurate guide to the glycemic index of sixty common foods, excerpted from the authoritative book *The Glucose Revolution*, coauthored by Jennie Brand-Miller, associate professor, University of Sydney, Australia, and Thomas M.S. Wolever, University of Toronto (Marlowe & Company, New York, 1999). The authors have conducted much of the research themselves and are regarded as international experts on the glycemic index. Their excellent book lists the glycemic indexes for three hundred foods. The book also contains numerous recipes with their glycemic index values, and explains how to figure glycemic indexes for your own recipes.

The better regulated your blood sugar and insulin, the better your brain is apt to work. For a steady supply of blood glucose, choose foods with the lower glycemic index number. If you occasionally want a quick spurt of blood glucose, you can choose foods with a high GI, such as dates or corn flakes.

FOOD	GLYCEMIC INDEX
Under 55: Low GI foods	
Between 55–70: Intermediate GI foods	
More than 70: High GI foods	
Angel food cake	67
Apple	38
Apple juice, unsweetened	40
Apricots, dried	31
Bagel	72
Baked beans	48
Banana	55
Beets, canned	64
Bread:	
French baguette	95
Sourdough	57
Whole wheat	69
White	70
Cereals:	
All Bran with extra fiber (Kellogg's)	51
Cheerios	74
Cocoa Puffs	77
Corn flakes	84
Oat bran	55
Bran flakes	74
Muesli, natural	56
Puffed wheat	80
Oatmeal, old fashioned	49
Raisin bran	73
Rice Chex	89
Total	76
Butter beans	31
Carrots, cooked	49
Bulgur	48
Corn, canned	55

FOOD	GLYCEMIC INDEX
Rice, instant	87
Rice, converted, Uncle Ben's	44
Rice, brown	55
Cherries	22
Chickpeas, canned	42
Chocolate bar	49
Cookie, vanilla wafer	77
Water cracker	78
Croissant	67
Milk, skim	32
Fettucine	32
French fries	75
Dates, dried	103
Grapefruit juice, unsweetened	48
Grapes	46
Orange	44
Orange juice	46
Pineapple	66
Raisins	64
Honey	58
Ice cream	61
Kidney beans	27
Lentils	30
Lima beans	32
Spaghetti, white, cooked	41
Peanuts	12
Popcorn	55
Potatoes, white-skinned, peeled, boiled	63
Potatoes, instant mashed	86
Potato chips	54
Pretzels	83
Soft drink	68

FOOD	GLYCEMIC INDEX
Soybeans	18
Sucrose	65
Yogurt, nonfat, fruit-flavored with sugar	33
Yogurt, nonfat, plain with artificial sweetener	14

Copyright Dr. Jennie Brand-Miller; reprinted with permission.

More Carbo Wisdom

In reality, you eat most foods in combination, not isolation, so the pure effect of high GI foods is usually blunted. Combining potatoes with low glycemic index foods, such as legumes, reduces the potato's glucose rush. Further, every individual is different, depending on internal controls on blood sugar. Therefore, it's difficult to know the ups and downs of your blood glucose unless you monitor it regularly. But you can make some very intelligent choices to try to keep blood sugar on an even keel if you know the correct glycemic index of various carbohydrate foods.

The type of carbohydrate you eat helps determine the levels and stability of your blood sugar. So does the amount, and foods vary greatly in carbohydrate content. For example, a half cup of carrots has only 3 grams of carbohydrates; a cup of cooked macaroni, 52 grams; 2 cups of popcorn, 12 grams; a plum, 7 grams.

Vinegar as Brain Food

Surprisingly, recent research finds that acidic foods, such as vinegar, can help save your brain from spikes in blood sugar. One Italian study showed that adding only four teaspoons of vinegar (part of a vinaigrette dressing also containing two teaspoons of oil) to an average meal depressed blood sugar by as much as 30 percent! Combining vinegar with high GI white potatoes, as in making potato salad, reduced the glycemic index 25 percent, according to tests by Jennie Brand-Miller, associate professor of nutrition at the University of Sydney in Australia. She found all types of vinegar, as well as lemon juice, effective, with red wine vinegar most potent. The explanation: The acid in some foods slows the digestive process or "gastric emptying rate," curtailing rapid rises in blood sugar.

Acidity also explains why sourdough bread has a very low GI compared with other breads; its yeast culture starter induces fermentation, releasing lactic acid. Yogurt also may help keep a lid on blood sugar, because it, too, contains lactic acid. Drinking grapefruit and orange juice may also lessen the impact of high glycemic foods, but not as much as vinegar. The reason: Small molecular weight acids, such as acetic (in vinegar) and lactic (in sourdough and yogurt), slow gastric emptying more than large molecular weight acids, such as citric and malic acids in citrus fruits.

Olive Oil as Brain Food

While you're at it, be sure to make your salad dressing with olive oil. New Australian research finds that olive oil and other monounsaturated fats promote higher good-type HDL cholesterol in diabetics, even when they eat lots of "fast" blood-sugar-raising carbohydrates. Olive oil somehow blunts the HDL-destroying powers of high glycemic index carbs. HDLs were also high in the study subjects when they ate a low glycemic index diet.

Ten Ways to Keep Blood Sugar Steady

- Know that starches, such as white potatoes and rice, can raise blood sugar faster and higher than eating sugar or candy. However, rice differs. Sticky cooked rice where grains clump together has a high GI. Basmati rice, where grains separate when cooked, has a low GI. Both brown rice and pasta have GIs similar to white rice and pasta. It's also a myth that pasta has a high GI and makes you fat. All pastas are fairly low GI foods, helping dampen blood sugar, appetite, and tendency to gain weight.

- Eat legumes with abandon. All legumes are slowly digested, causing slow, gradual rises in blood sugar, and thus have low GI ratings ranging from 48 to 18. This includes baked beans, butter beans, chickpeas, kidney beans, lentils, navy beans, soybeans, and peanuts, which technically are a legume and not a nut.

- If you eat high GI foods, combine them with low GI foods. That reduces the overall GI of a meal. Combining dried beans and rice, for example, produces an intermediate GI. When you eat snacks alone, choose ones with a low GI, such as apples, peanuts, popcorn. A high GI food, such as jelly beans eaten alone, is sure to spike blood sugar.

- Eat lots of vegetables and nuts. You can think of salad vegetables, such as carrots, tomatoes, onions, cucumbers, lettuce, broccoli, avocado, as well as nuts as "free" foods, with no significant impact on blood sugar. Their GI is effectively "zero" says Dr. Brand-Miller. Meat does not raise blood sugar, but its fat promotes insulin resistance. It's important to restrict high fat foods as well as high GI foods, she cautions, although lean meat can be nutritious.

- Restrict processed foods made with finely ground flour, such as bread, cereals, cookies, crackers. They have a high GI because the fine particles of starch zip right through your digestive tract. Many cereals and both white and whole wheat bread made from highly processed flour have higher GIs than table sugar, which has a GI of 60–65. White or whole wheat bread has a GI of 70. Most cold cereals have high GIs, above 70. Some with a low GI: AllBran with extra fiber, Bran Buds with psyllium, Special K, muesli.

- Add vinegar or lemon juice to foods to lower their glycemic index. Studies show that eating only four teaspoons of vinegar in a salad dressing with an average meal lowered blood sugar as much as 30 percent. Dr. Brand-Miller advises eating a salad with a vinegar or lemon juice dressing with high GI meals.

- Eat small amounts frequently. It's better for maintaining steady blood glucose if you eat several smaller meals six times a day rather than three times a day. It's the evolutionary thing to do also. "Our bodies were designed to eat little and often," says Dr. Benton.

- Be sure to eat something for breakfast. Overnight blood sugar levels sink and need replenishing. Your memory and learning abilities suffer if you don't feed your brain when it wakes up. Some experts favor a combination carbohydrate-protein breakfast, such as cereal with skim milk. Avoid pure carbohydrates (toast and jelly), pure proteins, and high animal fats.

- Take alpha-lipoic acid, a supplement that tends to lower blood sugar. Recommended dose for normal individuals: 50 to 100 milligrams a day. For diabetics: 300 to 600 milligrams daily.

- Take chromium supplements—200 micrograms if you are nondiabetic and 1000 micrograms if you are diabetic. U.S. Department of Agriculture researcher and diabetes specialist Dr. Richard Anderson finds that chromium tends to "normalize" blood sugar, bringing it up if it's low and down if it's high.

THE BEST AND THE WORST

Here is a capsule look at common foods with high and low glycemic index values, according to the latest Australian research. Best are those with low glycemic index values.

Food:	Low GI (slowly digested)	High GI (quickly digested)
Bread:	Sourdough (52)	French baguette (95)
Hot Cereal:	Oats, old (49) fashioned	Oats quick (65)
Cold Cereal:	Muesli (43) All Bran (51)	Corn flakes (84)
Dried Fruit:	Apricots (31)	Dates (103)
Fresh Fruit:	Cherries(22)	Watermelon (72)
Vegetable:	Sweet potato (54)	Red skin potato (93)
Grains:	Pasta, fettucine (32)	Instant rice (87)
Dairy Products:	Yogurt, fat free (14) fruit flavored with sugar (33)	Ice cream (61)
Candy:	M&M Peanuts (33)	Jelly beans (80)
Snacks:	Peanuts (14)	Pretzels (83)

Copyright Dr. Jennie Brand-Miller. Reprinted from *The Glucose Revolution* with permission.

How Sugar Can "AGE" Your Brain

There's another peculiar, and startling, hazard connected with high blood sugar that most people are quite unaware of, and it has serious implications for increased degenerative brain diseases, including Alzheimer's. High levels of blood sugar can make your entire body, including your brain, age faster, which is hardly a happy thought. In short, high circulating levels of blood sugar, as well as eating lots of sugar, can harm your brain by accelerating the aging process through chemical reactions in cells.

Leading expert Anthony Cerami at the Picower Institute for Medical Research in Manhasset, New York, explains that glucose in the blood reacts with proteins to create aberrant so-called "glycated or cross-linked proteins"—a kind of cellular debris that accumulates in cells, mucking up their mechanisms. These sugar-damaged proteins turn yellowish-brown, and are also called AGEs (advanced glycosylation end products), which is appropriate because they accelerate aging. They cause bones to "yellow," joints to stiffen, blood vessels to toughen and become clogged, and organs, including the brain, to malfunction. The process, says Dr. Cerami, resembles what happens to a chicken when you roast it in the oven. Its skin gets browned and crispy. We, too, are undergoing this "browning process" at body temperature as we age. "Basically, we are cooking very slowly over our lifetime," he says. In nerve cells, this browning process is not pretty.

These AGEs are just as dangerous to the brain as damage from oxygen-free radicals. In fact, AGEs compound their destruction by generating free radicals.

Researchers trying to solve the mysteries of human aging have known about AGEs for some time, and mainly blamed them on circulating levels of glucose in the blood—the higher the glucose, the greater the production of AGEs.

The sugar-damaged proteins are extremely high in the blood of diabetics, for example. Indeed, German researchers say that AGEs are the first step leading to diabetic nerve damage known as neuropathy. Researchers also believe this "glycation" process is a culprit in the destruction of brain cells leading to neurodegenerative diseases, including Alzheimer's, and possibly even in age-related memory loss.

A leading researcher, Siegfried Hoyer at the University of Heidelberg, proposes that some forms of Alzheimer's are tied to abnormalities in the way the brain metabolizes glucose, resulting in the overproduction of nerve-damaging AGEs, free radicals, and the formation of neurofibrillary tangles that kill off brain cells.

Caution: Sugar May Damage Brain Cells

What's new and alarming is that some researchers now say the risk of creating these destructive AGEs rises from consistently eating a diet high in simple sugars, independent of the blood glucose rises triggered by sugar intake. Roger B. McDonald, at the University of California at Davis, first showed that rats fed sucrose (ordinary table sugar) for most of their lives have shorter lifespans than rats fed comparable calories in starchy carbohydrates. In searching for the reason, he found that a high-sucrose diet created more AGEs. Indeed, he noted that the sucrose consumed, not blood glucose levels, mainly determined how many destructive AGEs were created.

In other animal studies, Israeli researchers discovered that eating excessive fructose may be even worse than eating sucrose or glucose. In a recent study, rats feasting on fructose showed the most damage from the sugar-protein reactions compared with those on high-sucrose or glucose diets. This is especially bad news, because in the last few decades consumption of fructose has skyrocketed, mainly due to the widespread use of high-fructose corn syrups in processed foods. Such fructose is used to sweeten soft drinks. That alone gives fructose extensive access to human brains, including young formative brains.

According to the Center for Science in the Public Interest, in 1996 the average American drank over 53 gallons of soft drinks!—up 43 percent since 1985. That's compared with twelve gallons of fruit juices and twenty-seven gallons of milk. A twelve-ounce can of non-diet cola boasts ten teaspoons of sugar, usually in the form of high-fructose corn syrup, and 150 calories. Although the use of artificial non-caloric sweeteners is also way up in recent years, sugar is still the primary sweetener by far.

Important antidotes: You can reduce sugar-inspired brain-damaging "glycation" by taking the supplement alpha-lipoic acid, says Dr. Lester Packer at the University of California at Berkeley. That's one reason lipoic acid seems to help prevent the onset of diabetes and its complications, notably neuropathy, he says. Recommended dose for diabetics: from 300 to 600 milligrams of alpha-lipoic acid daily.

Dr. Cerami has also recently discovered that alcohol partially blocks the AGE formation. AGEs dropped 52 percent in diabetic rats given some alcohol daily for four weeks compared with rats not given alcohol. Dr. Cerami surmises this is one reason drinking some alcohol reduces risk of cardiovascular disease.

BOTTOM LINE: *High blood levels of glucose as well as high intakes of sugar and fructose may lead to sugar-damaged proteins and nerve destruction. Remember: The brain was not designed to accommodate such consistent overloads of modern sugary foods and, understandably, may react badly.*

Chromium as Brain Food

Skimping on chromium could put you in the doldrums and steal your memory. A reason: Chromium helps regulate blood glucose. Indeed, a chromium deficiency in some individuals fosters impaired glucose tolerance and decreased number of insulin receptors (needed to process blood sugar), hypoglycemia, as well as high cholesterol and triglycerides.

Dr. Richard Anderson at the U.S. Department of Agriculture says chromium tends to normalize blood sugar—raising or lowering it, as needed. His research showed that 1000 daily micrograms of chromium reversed glucose intolerance and symptoms of diabetes. He recommends 200 micrograms of chromium daily to normalize blood sugar and prevent insulin resistance and diabetes in healthy adults.

Larry Christensen, Ph.D., chair of the psychology department at the University of South Alabama, says that people with major depression often have disturbances in processing glucose and consequently have exaggerated glucose responses, twice that of normal people. They also often have a marginal chromium deficiency. He says this chromium lack is compounded by the fact such persons often eat lots of sugar, perhaps in efforts to reverse their depression. But sugar depletes chromium, perpetuating a vicious circle that actually promotes depression.

In double-blind studies, Dr. Christensen found that a long-time high-sugar diet could promote persistent fatigue and depression in some people. In some individuals, he says, eating sugar creates a vicious cycle of mood swings, with a temporary burst of good feeling, followed by a downswing as blood sugar and the brain chemical serotonin fall. To raise their spirits they load up on more sugar, which again, after dives and rebounds in their blood sugar, makes them feel worse. The only long-term solution: Eat sugar sparingly or not at all to smooth out the sugar-inspired roller-coaster moods, advises Dr. Christensen. Taking chromium may also help.

HOW A HIGH-SUGAR DIET CAN BE BAD FOR YOUNG BRAINS

- Sugar replaces high vitamin and mineral foods, creating a deficit in nutrients the brain needs to function optimally.
- Some studies find that kids on high-sugar diets do worse on IQ tests, get poorer grades, and have more mood swings.
- Certain children, such as those with attention deficit disorder and hyperactivity, are often super-sensitive to high sugar intakes. PET scans show their brains do not burn glucose as efficiently. High blood sugar stimulates a greater release of cortisol—the "fight or flight" hormone—in such children.
- A chronic high intake of refined sugar at an early age is associated with poor attention spans in both normal and hyperactive children.
- High intakes of simple sugars, found in soft drinks and other processed foods, cause cellular damage (AGEs or glycation) in animals, known to promote nerve damage, premature aging in animals, and possibly degenerative brain diseases including Alzheimer's.

Since chromium can help alleviate poor glucose control that impairs mental function, it's definitely a "brain-boosting" nutrient.

BOTTOM LINE: *Try to keep blood glucose at normal levels for both good intellectual function and good moods. Best way to do that: Eat in ways compatible with your brain's evolutionary desires—choose low glycemic index carbohydrates that gradually raise blood glucose, making it steadily available to your brain. Cut back on sugar that may independently undermine good mental functioning and damage brain cells.*

How Antioxidants Make You Smart, Happy, and Save Your Brain from Aging

It's a scientific message of great urgency: One of the best things you can do for your brain is eat antioxidants. Antioxidants are universally recognized as the saviors of cells at all ages and under virtually all circumstances of health or disease. Antioxidants are chemicals that neutralize other hazardous chemicals called oxygen-free radicals that perpetually attack and damage bodily cells, disrupting their functioning and promoting aging and diseases of all kinds.

Scientists increasingly recognize that many mental problems from conception to death stem from too many rampaging free radicals and not enough antioxidants. In short, hordes of oxygen free radical thugs can get out of control, corrupting cells' genetic DNA, ripping their membranes, eroding their normal functioning, and sometimes destroying them. If you have a strong internal police force of antioxidants on patrol, the extent of the free radical damage to cells is limited.

You cannot avoid free radicals altogether. They are normal, in fact are generated when you breathe, or burn calories and glucose during normal metabolism. They also get in your body through cigarette smoke, air pollution, and toxic chemicals in the air and water. They also are carried into cells in foods, notably fatty foods. Under certain circumstances, they are good guys. For example, free radicals help destroy invading bacteria and viruses. But in general, they are the dark forces that attack fatty cell membranes and genetic material (DNA), creating permanent cellular damage that accumulates over time, leading to accelerated aging and virtually every chronic disease imaginable, including heart disease, cancer, diabetes, arthritis, and degenerative brain problems.

Thus, all your organs and tissues are subject to free radical assaults. But the brain appears to suffer most of all.

No question, free radicals are your brain's most malicious enemies. Your brain is the most vulnerable target of free radicals, say experts. One reason is that the brain generates more free radicals than other bodily tissue, because it uses so much oxygen and is the fattiest organ in the body. Fat is the favorite breeding ground for free radicals. Oxygen reacts with fat molecules in ways that generate free radicals—a process called oxidation—which leaves the fat oxidized or, in a word, rancid. A rancid brain is not a well-functioning brain. Indeed, the process in which the fat in brain cell membranes becomes oxidized, or rancid, occurs in many neurodegenerative conditions, such as Alzheimer's and Parkinson's. Rancid fat in brain cell membranes causes incredible havoc, screwing up release and uptake of neurotransmitters and transport of all-important glucose. Worse, oxidized fat cripples the functions of mitochondria (energy factories of cells), prompting a cascade of events that can cause cell death. The brain is also rich in iron, which sparks the formation of free radicals and fat oxidation.

How Free Radicals Destroy Your Brain

To keep the body alive, nature, in its evolutionary wisdom, devised a kind of SWAT team or antioxidant defense system to extinguish and dispose of the dangerous free radicals. Now, if you don't disarm these molecules, they entice certain cells in your body to actually self-destruct or commit suicide, a process called apoptosis; researchers believe that's what happens to destroy brain cells diseased with Alzheimer's.

> *"Your brain is particularly vulnerable to free radical damage for two reasons. First, it is a hotbed of activity; it never stops working. Brain cells need a constant flow of blood and oxygen to produce energy, which increases the production of free radicals. Second, the brain is composed of 50 percent fat, which makes it vulnerable to lipid peroxidation."* —Dr. Lester Packer, University of California, Berkeley

If you think of free radicals as thugs assaulting the cells of your brain and body, you can visualize the antioxidants as the body's ever-vigilant police force that searches out and destroys free radicals and attempts to repair their damage. Antioxidants vary in their ability to combat free radicals, but the stronger and more efficient they are, the greater their so-called "antioxidant capacity."

Generally, antioxidants do an admirable job, depending on their magnitude and efficiency. According to leading authority Bruce Ames, of the University of California at Berkeley, the DNA of a single cell takes about ten thousand

IF YOUR BRAIN GOES RANCID

The first step in the destruction of a nerve cell is often a process called "lipid peroxidation." It's the same event that turns LDL cholesterol particles toxic so they can infiltrate blood vessel walls, leading to a buildup of plaque and clogged arteries. It happens when unstable renegade "oxygen free radical" chemicals attack unsaturated fatty molecules in a cell's membranes. During the hit, the attackers leave the fat spoiled and rancid, crippling the cell so it can no longer properly move calcium out of the cell and glucose into the cell. Calcium can rise to toxic levels, initiating a cascade of events that activates poisonous glutamate and generates more free radicals as well as arachidonic acid, a nerve poison. It ends when the cell's command center, the mitochondria, dispatches "suicide proteins" and signals enzymes to depolarize inner membranes. In a fit of self-destruction, the cell's DNA disintegrates and it shrinks into oblivion. Another brain cell vanishes, and if enough are destroyed, the brain grows weaker and dysfunctional.

What's important about this process—which happens during normal aging as well as in degenerative brain diseases—is that you can stifle the initiating event, the lipid peroxidation of the cell's membrane, by getting specific fat-active antioxidants into your brain. Best at combating this lipid peroxidation of brain cells: vitamin E, lipoic acid, coenzyme Q10, flavonoids in fruits and vegetables. Also critical is glutathione, made internally by the body. But don't take glutathione supplements; they may encourage lipid peroxidation. Best way to raise glutathione in nerve cells: Take lipoic acid and vitamin C.

free radical hits per day. That's one cell. If you multiply that by trillions of cells, you can begin to visualize the potential extent of bodily devastation. However, antioxidants manage to repair at least 99 percent of the free radical damage to cells. Still, the tiny fraction of cellular damage that is not repaired accumulates over the years and eventually can cripple and destroy cells and shut down whole organs. Such cumulative damage from free radicals is a primary cause of premature aging, and age-related chronic diseases and disorders. Nowhere is the damage more tragic to the personality and intellect than in the brain. Of all major organs, at least in lab animals, the brain contains the lowest "antioxidant capacity," according to brain tissue analyses by Tufts University researchers. That is why it is all-important to maintain a highly efficient, functioning antioxidant defense system and to feed your brain a steady supply of antioxidants.

> **BOTTOM LINE:** *Your brain is the number one target of destructive "free radical" chemicals that rampage through your body, damaging cells and inducing premature aging, brain dysfunction, and virtually all other chronic diseases.*
>
> *The brain may be particularly vulnerable to the damaging effects of free radicals because it is relatively deficient in antioxidants to begin with."* —James Joseph, Ph.D., chief of neuroscience at the U.S. Department of Agriculture Human Nutrition Research Center on Aging at Tufts University

Deadly Imbalance

Every instant of your existence is an elegant dance of life and death between free radicals and antioxidants. When free radical activity gets the upper hand over antioxidant

activity, the result is an imbalance known in scientific jar-
gon as "oxidative stress." This means the free radical thugs
can overpower the antioxidant police and beat up on your
cells, causing their membranes to leak, their neuronal connections or dendrites and synapses to shrink, their energy
to be depleted, possibly ending in cell death. It's critical to
keep the right amounts of the right combination of antioxidants in your body and particularly in your brain. If free
radicals predominate, your brain is headed for trouble. If
antioxidants predominate, your brain is apt to stay in good
shape. Unfortunately, as you age, your body tends to produce more free radicals and fewer antioxidants, slowly tip-
ping the scales toward mental and physical decline. This
antioxidant production slowdown begins around age
twenty-five. That's why it is especially imperative to take in
more antioxidants as you get older, to try to maintain a
more youthful balance.

The Super "Network" Forces

Antioxidants are not like Lone Rangers with silver bullets,
working in isolation and independence. They are more like
small squads of soldiers that work together in exquisite
synchronized fashion to attack and disarm a common
enemy, the free radicals. They constantly talk to each other
and coordinate their survival. If one antioxidant exhausts
itself battling a free radical, another antioxidant often
rushes over to revive it. That remarkable discovery is fairly
new. Until a few years ago, researchers thought antioxidants worked independently. It's now known they are team
players. Dr. Lester Packer, professor of molecular and cell
biology at the University of California at Berkeley, has
developed the concept of an "antioxidant network," a
breakthrough in understanding how antioxidants work
together to provide full antioxidant protection.

Chemically, what happens when an antioxidant meets a free radical is surprising. In order to disarm or "quench" a free radical, an antioxidant merges with the free radical by donating an electron. That causes the antioxidant to become unstable and actually assume the characteristics of a relatively weak and harmless free radical, which then decomposes. Luckily, some exhausted antioxidants can be quickly rehabilitated—converted back to their original antioxidant form—when other antioxidants donate electrons needed for the transformation back. That's how certain antioxidants work together to revitalize each other in the heat of battle. For example, Dr. Packer explains, if vitamin E goes down while disarming a free radical, vitamin C or coenzyme Q10 can donate electrons, bringing vitamin E back to life as an antioxidant. The purpose, obviously, is to guarantee the survival of an all-important network of antioxidants in the body; otherwise, to stave off the hoards of free radicals created every microsecond, we would have to eat and synthesize incredible numbers of antioxidants.

However, only certain antioxidants have these special resuscitation talents, says Dr. Packer. He singles out five superstar antioxidants that make up the antioxidant network. They are vitamin E, vitamin C, glutathione, coenzyme Q10, and lipoic acid. These, he says, are the body's special forces, although many other chemicals in food and synthesized by the body are also antioxidants. Among the super five, only lipoic acid can resuscitate all the other network antioxidants, plus itself.

Antioxidants Tell Genes What to Do

Another recent exciting discovery is that antioxidants can help determine whether certain genes you possess are activated to cause mischief, including brain diseases. Frequently, you hear that genes have been linked to a disease or disorder, including ALS (Lou Gehrig's disease), Alzheimer's, Parkinson's, and Huntington's disease, as well as various cancers, arthritis, diabetes, cardiovascular disease. It seems that virtually every disorder may have a genetic component.

What many people do not realize is that having the gene does not mean it gets "expressed" or turned on. A gene is not destiny! A gene may not instigate trouble, unless it is prodded to do so. Scientists now know certain factors trigger activation of disease-related genes. A big one: free radicals. Thus, if a free radical or other hazard does not make a hit on a cell's genetic material, the gene may remain dormant and harmless. This also means antioxidants are mighty deterrents of gene-inspired disorders, because they block free radicals from trespassing through the membrane of the nucleus into the secluded living space where the genes or DNA are located. If the free radical attackers can't reach the genes, they can't damage them, inciting them to create chaos. Thus, nothing happens, despite your genetic vulnerability. One of the most monumental things antioxidants do, scientists now understand, is protect genes from expressing themselves and triggering disease.

> **BOTTOM LINE:** *Antioxidants can save you from your susceptibility to genetic diseases, including brain diseases and disorders, by stopping the "expression" or activation of the disease-prone genes.*

How do scientists know neurological dysfunction is tied to free radical damage? They see it. They have documented that free radical activity is a central event in the brains of people who suffer from degenerative brain diseases, such as ALS, Parkinson's, and notably Alzheimer's.

When brain researchers at the University of Kentucky's

Sanders-Brown Center on Aging examine slices of Alzheimer's brains, they find extensive evidence of free radical activity. In one comparison of thirteen Alzheimer's brains with ten normal brains, researchers detected high levels of substances signifying lipid peroxidation, the telltale fingerprints of free radicals, in all regions of the Alzheimer's brains except one. Further, they observed increased antioxidant activity by powerful warrior enzymes such as catalase. Moreover, it was clear that the forces of antioxidant enzymes were most prevalent in the very areas where fat peroxidation of cells was the most fierce, suggesting the brain had ordered out all the available troops in a pathetic effort to fend off the vast destruction, but failed miserably—since extensive brain cell death was obvious.

Save Your Brain: Eat Fruits and Vegetables
Where do you get the antioxidants that fight off the free radicals that would destroy your brain? Nature provided an army of antioxidants in the food supply. Fruits and vegetables are full of antioxidants, including vitamins and other more exotic chemicals called carotenoids and polyphenols. The evidence is overwhelming that eating antioxidant-packed fruits and vegetables and/or taking antioxidant vitamins can protect against free-radical damage and consequent death and disease. People who eat the most fruits and vegetables generally have the lowest rates of cancer, high blood pressure, heart disease, rheumatoid arthritis, diabetes, and premature death. For example, it's well established that high consumption of fruits and vegetables can slash your risk of developing various cancers in half! Most scientists believe fruits and vegetables convey antioxidant activity that curbs cancer- and disease-inciting damage from free radicals.

Antioxidants, in a word, can slow the aging process of the entire body, and are particularly needed in the brain.

Only in the last ten years have scientists dissected fruits and vegetables in search of the magic chemicals (in addition to vitamins and minerals) that account for their monumental antioxidant activity. Many strong antioxidants have been identified. Among the so-called carotenoids are beta-carotene, alpha-carotene, lycopene, lutein, and xeazanthin. A huge family of some four thousand antioxidants known as flavonoids is concentrated in deeply colored fruits and vegetables and considered mainly responsible for their antioxidant activity. Pioneering scientists at the U.S. Department of Agriculture in Beltsville, Maryland, have analyzed many foods to find and quantify specific exotic antioxidants, such as lycopene in tomatoes and lutein in green leafy vegetables. So it's now possible to know how much of these powerful carotenoids is contained in which plant foods.

But in a ground-breaking step, agriculture researchers at Tufts University in Boston have developed a method of analyzing each food, not for its individual component antioxidants, but for its overall "antioxidant capacity." After blending up three samples of a specific food, such as spinach or strawberries from the supermarket, researchers put the pulp and extract through a "high performance liquid chromatograph"—a machine that analyzes how well and how quickly antioxidants in the sample food disarm free radicals, such as peroxyl and hydroxyl radicals, the type we make during normal metabolism. This test, says its developer, USDA research scientist Guohua (Howard) Cao, measures all traditional antioxidants, such as vitamin C, vitamin E, beta-carotene, and glutathione, and reveals a food's total antioxidant capacity, known as ORAC (oxygen radical absorbency capacity.) Thus, each food gets an ORAC score. An ORAC score signifies how well nature endowed that food with overall powers to neutralize cell-damaging free radicals. Highest are fruits and vegetables.

It's no longer just how much antioxidant beta-carotene or lycopene or anthocyanins a food has. What really counts is the total antioxidant amount it provides.

At the top of the list of antioxidant powerhouses, as judged by the ORAC test: prunes, raisins, blueberries, blackberries, garlic, kale, cranberries, strawberries, spinach, raspberries—generally fruits and vegetables with the deepest colors—as well as tea and red wine. Dr. Cao explains that the pigment itself is a potent antioxidant. Experts also know that the total antioxidant capacity of a food may be far greater than the sum of its individual antioxidant components. Fruits and vegetables contain a complex assortment of countless antioxidants that interact and potentiate each other, pushing their antioxidant powers far above their mere additive value. The ORAC test accounts for that synergism.

The Best Brain-Saving Fruits and Vegetables
According to tests at Tufts University, here's how fifty-three fruits and vegetables rank on antioxidant capacity (ORAC)—ability to fight off free radical chemicals that attack your brain cells.

SUPER ANTIOXIDANT FRUITS
AND VEGETABLES

ORAC Units

	per 100 grams		*per item or serving*	
1. Prunes	5770	1 pitted prune	462
2. Raisins	2830	1/4 cup	1019
3. Blueberries	2234	1/2 cup	1620
4. Blackberries	2036	1/2 cup	1466
5. Garlic	1939	1 clove	58
6. Kale	1770	1/2 cup ckd	1150
7. Cranberries	1750	1/2 cup	831
8. Strawberries	1536	1/2 cup	1144
9. Spinach, raw	1210	1 cup	678
10. Raspberry	1227	1/2 cup	755
11. Brussels sprouts	981	1 sprout	206
12. Plum	949	1 plum	626
13. Alfalfa sprouts	931	1 cup	307
14. Spinach, steamed	909	1/2 cup ckd	1089
15. Broccoli florets	888	1/2 cup ckd	817
16. Beets	841	1/2 cup ckd, sliced	715
17. Avocado	782	1/2 Florida	149
18. Orange	750	1 orange	982
19. Grape, red	739	10 grapes	177
20. Pepper, red	731	1 med pepper	540
21. Cherry	670	10 cherries	455
22. Kiwifruit	602	1 fruit	458
23. Beans, baked	503	1/2 cup	640
24. Grapefruit, pink	483	1/2 fruit	580
25. Beans, kidney	460	1/2 cup ckd	400
26. Onion	449	1/2 cup chopped	360
27. Grapes, white	446	10 grapes	107
28. Corn	402	1/2 cup ckd	330

ORAC Units

per 100 grams		per item or serving	
29. Eggplant	386	1/2 cup ckd	185
30. Cauliflower	377	1/2 cup ckd	234
		1/2 cup raw	188
31. Peas, frozen	364	1/2 cup ckd	291
32. Potatoes	313	1/2 cup cooked	244
33. Potatoes, sweet	301	1/2 cup cooked	301
34. Cabbage	298	1/2 cup raw	105
35. Leaf lettuce	262	10 leaves	200
36. Cantaloupe	252	1/2 melon	670
37. Banana	221	1 banana	252
38. Apple	218	1 med apple	300
39. Tofu	213	1/2 cup	195
40. Carrots	207	1/2 cup raw	115
		1/2 cup ckd	160
41. Beans, string	201	1/2 cup ckd	125
42. Tomato	189	1 med	233
43. Zucchini	176	1/2 cup raw	115
44. Apricots	164	3 raw	175
45. Peach	158	1 med	137
46. Squash, yellow	150	1/2 cup ckd	183
47. Beans, lima	136	1/2 cup	115
48. Lettuce, iceberg	116	5 large leaves	116
49. Pear	134	1 med	222
50. Watermelon	104	1/16 th 10" diam	501
51. Melon, honeydew	97	1/10 melon	125
52. Celery	61	1/2 cup diced	60
53. Cucumber	54	1/2 cup slices	28

Calories and Antioxidants

Why do prunes and raisins rank so high in antioxidant capacity? Because drying removes water and concentrates their antioxidants. Plums, which become prunes when dried, have only 16 percent as much ORAC value. It's the same for grapes, which become raisins. Thus, dried fruits are an efficient way to get antioxidants into your body, although they carry a liability of a few extra calories. When you eat 3240 ORACs in a cup of blueberries you take in 82 calories; the same number of ORACs in seven prunes gives you 140 calories. The best way to get scads of antioxidant power with minuscule calories: drink tea.

Super Brain-Saving Juices

You can't always judge a juice by its source. Tests show that commercial grape juice and tomato juice had much higher antioxidant capacity than fresh red grapes and fresh tomatoes. But commercial orange juice had lower antioxidant capacity than fresh oranges. Incidentally, red wine had about the same antioxidant capacity as red grape juice.

Of five juices tested in Tufts labs, red grape juice (Welch's 100% Concord) won by a mile! It has four times more antioxidant capacity than the others. Unfortunately, it is also high in sugar. Grapefruit, tomato, and orange were approximately equal in antioxidant activity, with apple juice less so.

Turn Yourself into an Antioxidant

Think of it this way: Your whole body is exposed to constant assaults by free radical chemicals that, to be blunt, tend to turn you and your brain rancid, just like a piece of fatty meat out of the refrigerator too long. But what if you could don a kind of internal Superman suit that acts as armor to repel or neutralize those perpetual chemical attacks? Actually, you can. That's what fortifying yourself with antioxidants really does. Scientists now have good evidence that piling in antioxidants builds an invisible biological armor that helps deflect attacks on cells and on sensitive brain tissue in particular. You can become your own best antioxidant. Relatively new commercial blood tests can reveal how strong your antioxidant defenses are. (See page 173 for where to get such a blood test.)

Unquestionably, if you could check your blood after eating antioxidant-rich fruits and vegetables, it would show that the antioxidants are digested and absorbed. Most important, scientists have proof that eating antioxidant-rich foods boosts antioxidant protection, as measured by the ORAC test. Tufts researchers Drs. Ronald L. Prior and Guohua Cao tested the antioxidant capacity of the blood of thirty-six normal healthy men and women, ages twenty to eighty. In the year before the study began, the subjects averaged five servings of fruits and vegetables daily, containing 1670 ORAC units. During the fifteen-day test, they doubled consumption to ten daily servings, and 3300–3500 ORAC units daily. The exciting part: This and subsequent experiments showed that blood antioxidant capacity jumped 15 to 25 percent.

Interestingly, Drs. Prior and Cao found that the antioxidant capacity of humans may plateau, so that adding more fruits and vegetables does not always push it up farther.

How much it takes to elevate antioxidant activity and how high you can drive it up depends on individual makeup. Dr. Cao explains that each person has a distinctive internal antioxidant defense system, and how much you can improve it by eating more fruits and vegetables depends on your unique biology. If your antioxidant defenses are low, you may get a bigger boost than someone with an existing high-antioxidant capacity, he says. "Each body regulates antioxidant defenses, depending on a multitude of factors, including genes."

How Much Is Enough?

According to Tufts tests, most Americans should eat more than 3500 ORAC units a day to significantly lift human antioxidant activity, says Dr. Prior. Eating 5000 to 6000 ORAC units daily would be more protective. Most Americans now take in about 1200 ORAC units daily, averaging about three fruits and vegetables per day, according to USDA estimates. The number of ORACS you take in daily, of course, depends on which fruits and vegetables you choose. As Dr. Prior says, "you can pick seven with low values and get only about 1300 ORAC units. Or you can eat seven with high values and reach 6000 ORAC units or more."

It's not difficult. One cup of blueberries alone provides 3200 ORAC units! Add ½ cup strawberries and an orange, and you're already up to 5500. Note: Fruit is generally higher in antioxidant capacity than vegetables.

The message is no longer just to eat fruits and vegetables; the information is now available to enable you to choose ones with the most powerful antioxidant capabilities to ward off cell deterioration.

BOTTOM LINE: *Eating fruits and vegetables is an easy way to make a dramatic impact in saving your brain cells from destruction. And you can do it rapidly— within several days! In young people antioxidant capacity rose dramatically in five to six days. People over age sixty needed ten to eleven days to reach the same heights of antioxidant capacity, according to Tufts tests.*

Eating ten ounces of fresh spinach pushed up blood antioxidant scores more than taking 1250 milligrams of vitamin C. Eight ounces of strawberries boosted blood antioxidants as much as drinking two five-ounce glasses of red wine.

Stop Brain Decline: Eat Spinach and Strawberries

As you age, the cells in your central nervous system may decline in function, even though you have no degenerative brain diseases such as Alzheimer's or Parkinson's. One possible reason: With age, the neurotransmitter receptors on cell membranes lose sensitivity, so they no longer process messages as efficiently. An underlying cause of that diminution in communication among cells appears to be both increased attacks by free radicals and a diminished supply of protective antioxidants. A research team headed by James A. Joseph at Tufts theorized that they might be able to block that normal age-related loss of brain function by feeding laboratory animals spinach, strawberries, or vitamin E to buck up antioxidant defenses. It was a stunning idea with a remarkable outcome and exciting implications.

The animals started eating four different diets (control or ordinary, spinach, strawberries, or vitamin E) at six months of age or about age twenty in human terms. They continued on the diets for eight months—into middle age. When the rats reached fifteen months (forty five to fifty years in human terms), an age when their memories were expected to decline, they were put through a battery of tests. One test, in which the animals paddle around a deep pool to find a submerged platform where they can rest, measures changes in long-term and short-term memory.

No question, animals fed spinach for about half their lifetimes showed superior long-term memory; they remembered where to find the hidden platforms much better than those fed the other diets, meaning the spinach-eaters retained more of their learning ability. Next best at boosting memory: strawberries.

To see if extraordinarily vigorous memory was reflected in brain cell biology, Dr. Joseph examined specific areas of the animals' brains, particularly the region that controls cognitive function—the neostriatum. Cells in this area become insensitive or sluggish in releasing chemical messengers, such as dopamine, as animals and humans age. In fact, by middle age, rats' striatal cells have lost about 40 percent of their ability to respond. And, not unexpectedly, this did happen in rats fed an ordinary "control diet."

But, amazingly, animals fed spinach, strawberries, and vitamin E did not lose such brain cell power; they released dopamine as they did when younger. They, indeed, scored twice as high in performance tests of their striatal brain cells as those on "control diets." Most effective of all in protecting brain cells in this aspect was spinach. The spinach-eating rodents also scored best in a test of nerve cells in the cerebellum, an area of the brain that controls balance and coordination.

For the first time, scientists proved that eating spinach and strawberries had a dramatic impact in averting the expected decline in brain function and memory that comes with age. Dr. Joseph credits the foods' long-term antioxidant activity that prevented brain cell damage. But he also notes that the flavonoids in the spinach and strawberries can also increase fluidity of brain cell membranes (like fish oil does), thus suggesting another way of blocking age-related brain deficits.

Of course, the big implication is that if spinach and strawberries work such miracles in the brains of small mammals, they will also do the same in the brains of large mammals, namely humans. How much spinach or strawberries did it take to prevent decline in brain function? Not much. The human equivalent of only a pint of strawberries a day or a large spinach salad. Dr. Joseph contends that "nutritional intervention with fruits and vegetables may play an important role in preventing the long-term effects of oxidative [free radical] stress on brain function."

Interestingly, vitamin E, a known strong antioxidant, had only a moderate effect in protecting animals' brains from decline. It was less effective than spinach or strawberries. Dr. Joseph speculates that the foods worked better because they possess multiple antioxidants that interact to produce a synergistic effect (a more potent effect combined than each alone).

> **BOTTOM LINE:** *To save your brain from disintegration, you need to eat lots of berries, spinach, and other deeply colored fruits and vegetables with high antioxidant activity.*

Rejuvenate Your Brain: Eat Blueberries

Next question: Can eating high-antioxidant fruits and vegetables also *reverse* brain cell damage, motor coordination malfunction and memory loss due to normal aging? Yes, finds Dr. Joseph.

Once your brain has experienced gradual dysfunction, perhaps even undetected, can you rejuvenate it? Can you actually reverse some of the decline? In short, can you repair the brain's broken circuits, restoring some of its lost functioning? Even Dr. Joseph was not totally surprised that strawberries and spinach prevented decline. But reversing such aging damage that had already occurred was another matter. He knew of nothing, outside maybe a strong experimental drug, that had ever done it or could be expected to do it. But he thought he would give it a shot.

Dr. Joseph decided to add blueberries this time. New USDA analyses had recently found blueberries to be an antioxidant superpower, better even than strawberries or spinach. The chosen rats were old—between 65 and 70 in human terms, with age-related brain deficits, resulting in diminished memory, motor coordination, and balance. For eight weeks, they were fed a regular control diet or diets containing 1 to 2 percent of calories from either extracts of fresh blueberries, strawberries, or spinach, processed into a freeze-dried powder and mixed with their regular chow.

At the end of the experiment, the animals were re-tested. The unthinkable had happened. All the rats eating the blueberries, strawberries, or spinach displayed better mental faculties than at the beginning of the experiment. In other words, their mental deficits had been dramatically reversed. Their brains were now functioning at much younger levels.

How much younger? How much did their brain deficits regress? "Well, some of them were as good as "young" and some were as good as "middle-age, at least middle-age." It's the damndest thing I ever saw," says an astounded Dr. Joseph.

In other words, you fixed the brain's machinery?

"Yes."

And how much did they have to eat in human terms?

"Only about half a cup of blueberries a day."

You're kidding.

"No, it's amazing."

All three—blueberries, spinach, and strawberries— improved short-term memory—of the type needed to remember phone numbers long enough to dial them. But only blueberries reversed deficits in coordination and balance. This is highly significant, because such motor coordination typically starts to decline by middle age, and there is no known way to prevent or reverse it. The fact that blueberries may do so is an exciting discovery. For example, aged rats are able to traverse a narrow rod for only five seconds before losing their balance and falling off. After eating blueberries for two months, they were able to stay on the rod more than twice as long—eleven seconds.

When Dr. Joseph looked further, he found more striking evidence of the blueberry phenomenon. Examinations of their brains clearly revealed concrete cellular changes related to their mental rejuvenation. He verified that the insensitivity of receptors in brain cells had been partly reversed. Thus, much of the eroded integrity of the brain's circuitry had been restored, accounting for their improved mental capacities.

Then, he decided to put blueberries to another test. He first exposed animal neurons to a toxic substance, known to cause extensive free radical damage in neurons, including dreaded calcium dysregulation that helps ruin human brain cells, inducing dementia. Sure enough, it was devastation. Then he took the damaged cells and poured blueberry extract over them. When he tested them again, the dementia-inducing toxicity had completely vanished, neutralized by the blueberries.

"Sure, I was surprised. I know of no other agent that could reverse motor behavioral and cognitive defects from aging. It's the only thing I have ever found that does it—and I have been searching for twenty-two years."

Other brain researchers, along with Dr. Joseph, are now testing the blueberry's powers to see if it can prevent or reverse Alzheimer's-like brain damage in animals.

Carotenoids on the Brain

There's plenty of evidence that what Tufts researchers found in animals happens in humans. Among 1400 older men and women, those with the highest blood levels of fruit and vegetable antioxidants called carotenoids (beta- and alpha-carotene, lutein, zeaxanthin, cryptoxanthin, and lycopene) were smarter, according to tests at the French government's medical research institute (INSERM). Individuals with the highest blood carotenoids, indicating they ate the most fruits and vegetables, scored 35 to 40 percent higher on tests of logical reasoning and visual attention than those with the lowest blood levels of carotenoids. Presumably, the high carotenoids produced stronger brain power by shielding brain cells from free radical damage due to aging.

Antioxidants Predict Memory

Similarly, Swiss researchers recently found that high blood levels of antioxidant vitamin C and beta-carotene actually *predicted* a superior memory in old age. In a large ongoing study of aging, Walter J. Perrig, Ph.D., and colleagues at the University of Berne recently tested the memory performance of 442 healthy men and women ages sixty-five to ninety-four. Dr. Perrig compared their memory scores with blood samples, taken recently and twenty-two years previously. Strikingly, those with the most blood vitamin C and beta-carotene, at both time periods, scored highest on tests of memory involving recall, recognition, and vocabulary. Thus, high blood antioxidants were an accurate forecast of memory strength two decades later. Researchers concluded that these antioxidants "play an important role in brain aging and . . . the prevention of progressive cognitive impairments." In short, if you want to preserve your memory as you get old, be sure to take in lots of antioxidants, vitamin C and beta-carotene in particular.

Tomatoes and the Nun Experiments

It's almost incredible that the amount of tomatoes you eat over a lifetime could help determine how vital your brain is in old age. But striking research by David Snowdon, M.D., at the Sanders-Brown Center on Aging at the University of Kentucky, says it's true. Dr. Snowdon is director of an ongoing study of aged nuns, many over a hundred years old. He has found that the more lycopene—a potent antioxidant—in their blood, the sharper their mental acuity in old age. Lycopene gets into the blood virtually only one way: from eating tomatoes.

In Dr. Snowdon's study of eighty eight women ages seventy-seven to ninety-eight, those with low blood lycopene were least able to take care of themselves in old age—least able to walk, bathe, dress, and feed themselves. Such women with a "lycopene deficiency" in fact were nearly four times more apt to require assistance than those with above average lycopene. Dr. Snowdon theorizes that antioxidant lycopene in tomatoes helps neutralize free radical chemicals throughout the body, including the brain, keeping it intact and functioning better and longer. Indeed low cognitive function, presumably related to free radical damage in the brain, strongly predicted a progressive loss of independence in activities of daily living.

Although watermelon and pink grapefruit contain smidgens of lycopene, by far the major source is the tomato, notably processed tomato products, such as tomato paste, tomato sauce, and canned tomatoes. A recent Italian study showed that eating tomato puree with 16.5 milligrams of lycopene daily for twenty-one days boosted the blood's antioxidant capacity dramatically. Free radical damage to cells' DNA (genetic material) dropped an astonishing 33 percent.

WHERE TO FIND BRAIN-SAVING LYCOPENE

	1 ounce
Tomato paste	16 mg
Tomato ketchup	5 mg
Spaghetti sauce	5 mg
Tomato sauce	5 mg
Tomatoes, canned	3 mg
Tomato soup	3 mg
Tomato juice	3 mg
Vegetable juice	3 mg
Watermelon	1 mg
Pink grapefruit	1 mg
Fresh tomatoes	less than 1 mg

Tea: The Thinking Human's Drink

Tea is an astonishing source of antioxidants. Drinking tea can soak your brain in antioxidants, potentially slowing down brain decline. There's evidence tea can cut the risk of stroke. A study of 6000 Japanese women found that those who drank at least five cups of green tea every day had half as many strokes as women who drank less. Dutch researchers found that older tea drinkers (a couple of cups a day) cut their odds of fatal heart disease in half. That implies that tea helped keep blood vessels healthy, microvessels that feed the brain as well as the heart. Other research shows that tea can thwart dreaded "lipid peroxidation" that first step to brain cell destruction.

Drs. Prior and Cao at Tufts have analyzed the antioxidant capacity of various types of teas on the market. The first surprise: Samples of *black* tea leaves on average had about 80 percent more antioxidant capacity than green tea leaves. However, some green tea was almost as high in

ORACs as the top black tea. Both black and green tea ranged widely in antioxidant capacity. Some researchers, notably in Japan, declare green tea superior because it has four times more of one specific antioxidant, epigallocatechin gallate (EGCG), than black tea. But overall, black tea ranks higher in total antioxidant potency, according to Tufts analyses.

The antioxidant capacity also depends on how long you brew tea. Tufts researchers put one black or green teabag in five ounces of boiling water. Within five minutes, about 85 percent of the tea bag's antioxidant potential was released. The other 15 percent was released after another five minutes of brewing. The finding: A five-ounce cup of black or green tea brewed five minutes provides on average 1246 ORAC units! That's right up there near spinach and strawberries, proved to delay brain decline in animals.

Inarguably, tea antioxidants do get into your bloodstream. One test by Italian researchers found that drinking a single cup of strong black or green tea revved up antioxidant activity in the blood by 41 to 48 percent. In this study, green tea produced peak antioxidant activity within thirty minutes, and black tea within fifty minutes. Antioxidants stayed elevated for about an hour and a half before returning to normal.

Tea Without Antioxidants

If you're looking for antioxidants to help your brain, forget instant (powdered) tea mixes, bottled teas, or herbal teas. They have little or no antioxidant activity, according to Tufts University analyses. Also, real tea with caffeine packs more antioxidant protection than decaffeinated tea. Tufts tests showed brewed decaffeinated tea contained about half the amount of antioxidants as regular brewed tea containing caffeine.

A recent Tufts analysis of twenty different herbal teas found only one with any significant antioxidant activity. Similarly, a few years ago, British researchers found no antioxidants in a couple of dozen herbal teas. Herbal teas may have some specific medicinal values, but you can't depend on them to help protect your brain or other cells against free radical assaults. If you want brain protection, drink the real stuff.

In other tests of tea's antioxidant properties, researcher Dr. Andrew Waterhouse at the University of California at Davis found that tea supplied as many antioxidants, known as catechins, as red wine. He found that a glass of red wine has 300 milligrams of catechins; a cup of green tea has 375 milligrams; and a cup of black tea contains 210 milligrams. Dr. Waterhouse says drinking tea provides as much antioxidant protection as red wine.

Iced tea can have just as much antioxidant value as hot tea if you brew tea bags or tea leaves—and then add ice. Instant ice tea mixes are a waste—totally devoid of antioxidants, according to Tufts analyses.

> **BOTTOM LINE:** *Drinking real tea (brewed from tea bags or leaves) is a quick, easy, calorie-free way to feed your brain antioxidants. Instant powdered teas, bottled teas, and herbal teas do not contain any significant antioxidant activity.*

Caution: Adding a couple of teaspoons of milk to a cup of tea may help release antioxidants, according to research by John Weisburger, Ph.D., of the American Health Foundation. But adding more milk is detrimental, tending to neutralize tea's antioxidants.

Chocolate as Brain Food

Surprising as it may seem, chocolate contains antioxidants that help protect the brain from aging and disease, as well as other psychoactive chemicals that make you feel good. In fact, Harvard researchers recently declared that people who eat chocolate live on average one year longer. The probable reason: chocolate's rich content of antioxidants.

In a recent chemical analysis of chocolate, the University of California's Dr. Waterhouse found that it contains polyphenols—the same class of antioxidants that are in red wine, tea, and fruits and vegetables. In fact, he deemed the phenols in chocolate more potent antioxidants than those in red wine, in some cases almost twice as potent. Dr. Waterhouse detected 205 milligrams of phenolics in an ounce-and-a-half chocolate bar—about the same as you get in a five-ounce glass of red wine. Two tablespoons of cocoa, typically used to make a cup of hot chocolate, has 145 mg of phenols. Dark chocolate has the most; white chocolate has none. Eating dark chocolate and drinking red wine together would boost antioxidant activity beyond that expected from simply adding the antioxidants of each, says Dr. Waterhouse.

Recent Japanese tests identified the precise antioxidants in cacao liquor, one of the major ingredients of chocolate, as various catechins, long known to be the active antioxidant agents in both green and black tea. In fact, Japanese researchers found that antioxidant polyphenols made up a remarkable 7 to 13 percent of cacao liquor obtained from several countries. This means, they said, that chocolate may guard against the awful "lipid peroxidation" that can warp and destroy the fatty membranes of brain cells as well turn blood fats toxic. Further tests showed that phenols extracted from chocolate did suppress free radical damage to cells in human blood samples.

Mind-Altering Drugs in Chocolate

Eating chocolate can also give your brain a mood-lifting fix. Chocolate is one of the most powerful mood elevators, says British research psychologist David Benton, Ph.D., at the University of Wales-Swansea. To prove it, he did studies in which he played dirge-type music that put students into a depressed mood. Then he offered them either milk chocolate or carob, a chocolate imitation. He found that choosing chocolate raised their moods. Also, their chocolate craving rose as their mood sank. The chocolate substitute, carob, did not work.

Dr. Benton says chocolate contains, in addition to serotonin-boosting sugar and mind-soothing fat, several pharmacologically active chemicals that stimulate the central nervous system including phenylethylamine, similar in some aspects to amphetamine, a well-known upper.

Moreover, researchers at the Neurosciences Institute in San Diego recently suggested another intriguing reason for chocolate's hold on the brain. Chocolate may have the same mind-soothing effects as marijuana. The researchers discovered that novel constituents in cocoa powder and chocolate are chemical cousins of anandamide which binds to the same receptors on brain cells as marijuana. This means chocolate chemicals may activate receptors for marijuana and thus mimic its psychoactive effects of heightened sensations and euphoria. If you got enough anandamide chemicals in your brain from eating chocolate, it might produce "a transient feeling of well-being," and help account for chocolate cravings, researchers concluded.

Other explanations for why chocolate is the most craved of all foods, notably by women: The sugar in chocolate foods boosts mood-elevating levels of the neurotransmitter serotonin. The fat boosts other "feel-good" brain chemicals called endorphins.

Chocolate may even have a stronger allure for brain cells than alcohol. In tests some animals tend to reduce their intake of alcohol when they are given a chocolate drink as an option.

Make It Red Wine

If you drink alcohol, research suggests the best choice is a daily glass of wine, preferably red wine with food. Red wine, but not white wine, is full of antioxidants that may help protect the brain from free-radical damage, strokes, and age-related memory loss. On the other hand, heavy drinking of any alcoholic beverage, including red wine, can kill brain cells, leading to brain atrophy, decline in cognitive functions, and dementia. Binge drinking is particularly damaging to the brain and more apt to trigger strokes. However, in moderation, alcohol is anti-inflammatory and tends to boost good HDL cholesterol, which may help save blood vessels from destruction. The major secret of red wine appears to be its high concentration of antioxidants that are lacking in other alcoholic beverages.

Among a large group of 3700 French men and women over age sixty-five, moderate drinkers of wine were only 18 percent as likely as nondrinkers to suffer severe intellectual decline with age (dementia). Such wine drinkers were only 25 percent as apt to develop Alzheimer's disease. The study was done by French researcher Jean Marc Orgogozo, M.D., head of neurology at the Hospital Pellegrin in Bordeaux. Previously, he had found that the same group of moderate wine drinkers performed better on a test of cognitive function than nondrinkers. Most wine consumed in France is red.

Danish investigators have recently found that moderate wine drinkers were at lower risk of stroke.

FIVE REASONS RED WINE IN MODERATION MAY BENEFIT THE BRAIN

Provides antioxidants: Red wine is exceptionally high in antioxidant polyphenols, particularly anthocyanins; white wine and dark beer also have some antioxidants; spirits such as vodka, gin, scotch, and whiskey have little or none. The antioxidants help protect brain cells from free-radical attacks, genetic damage, malfunction, and death.

Protects blood vessels: Alcohol raises good HDL cholesterol and slightly lowers bad LDL cholesterol. The antioxidant polyphenols in red wine act as anticoagulants, clot-dissolving agents and artery dilators. Thus, a glass of wine a day, notably with food, may reduce plaque buildup in carotid arteries and discourage clot-type strokes in cerebral vessels.

Fights inflammation: Alcohol itself has anti-inflammatory activity, important because inflammation in the brain contributes to blood vessel and brain cell destruction and possibly Alzheimer's disease.

Boosts estrogen: Wine raises levels of estrogen, which also is an antioxidant, thought to help protect against mental deterioration and Alzheimer's. Judith S. Gavaler, of the Oklahoma Medical Research Foundation, has found that plant hormones in alcoholic beverages induce estrogenic activity. Most potent is red wine. She showed that, after removing all alcohol, one glass of red wine triggered an estrogenic response in 92 percent of postmenopausal women; the figures were 83 percent for an ounce of bourbon and 77 percent for a can of beer or glass of white wine. More than one daily drink produced no greater estrogenic effect, indicating this may be the optimal dose, says Dr. Gavaler.

Blocks AGE formation: New evidence suggests that alcohol inhibits formation of damaging protein-sugar reactions in cells that accelerate cell aging, memory decline, and poor mental functioning, even brain disease and dementia.

Alcohol as Brain-Buster

Studies find that too much alcohol can damage the brain. One recent study at Indiana University School of Medicine found that elderly light drinkers (fewer than four drinks per week) scored slightly better on tests of thinking ability than nondrinkers. But those who drank ten or more drinks per week scored more poorly on the cognitive tests than nondrinkers.

Note: You don't need alcohol to get antioxidant benefits from beverages. Purple grape juice and tea can give you as much as red wine—without the alcohol.

The Carnivore Connection

Whether you are a vegetarian or meat-eater also can rig the chances of becoming demented or "senile" later in life. In fact, eating meat may more than double your odds of eventually becoming demented, compared with being a strict vegetarian. That's what researchers at Loma Linda University School of Medicine found when they studied 272 California residents as part of a Seventh Day Adventist study. Definitely, there was a delayed onset of dementia in vegetarians. Why? Does meat inflict harm on the brain or do the high quantities of vegetables convey special brain protection, presumably by acting as antioxidants? Probably both.

Meat contains both high amounts of saturated fat and iron that can damage brain cells. It's well established that iron acts as a catalyst in promoting generation of brain damaging free-radical chemicals. Consuming excessive iron and meat is blamed for contributing to other free radical diseases—heart disease and cancer. It seems likely the same iron- and meat-inspired free-radical bombardment of the brain promotes cellular damage that is manifested as dementia.

> **BOTTOM LINE:** *One of the most important actions you can take to save your brain from gradual deterioration that may start in your twenties is to eat a diet rich in various antioxidants. And it appears it's never too early or too late to start. Eating antioxidants even late in life might help reverse mental decline that has already occurred.*

How Calories Steal Your Brain

Everybody knows that overeating can pack on pounds that strain your heart. But the fact that excessive calories are also extremely hazardous to your brain is largely unknown. As Americans grow ever more overweight, so does the prospect of impending brain damage from ordinary aging, as well as Alzheimer's and Parkinson's disease, say scientists. Today's epidemic of obesity could well become an epidemic of brain degeneration in the years ahead, says neurobiologist Mark Mattson, Ph.D., a leading brain researcher at the University of Kentucky Sanders-Brown Center on Aging. He sees cutting down on calories as one of the most effective things

---

DO YOU HAVE AN ANTIOXIDANT DEFICIENCY?

One way to find out whether your brain is being deprived of protective antioxidants is to have your blood tested. That test will reveal your levels of various antioxidants, including vitamins E and C, as well as lycopene and coenzyme Q10, in comparison with others of your age and gender. It will provide an antioxidant profile in percentiles for the important antioxidants in your blood, thus telling you whether you are eating enough fruits and vegetables and/or taking adequate supplements.

One lab highly recommended by antioxidant researcher Dr. Lester Packer is Pantox. You can contact them at 1–888–726–8698 or through their web site: http://www.pantox.com.

The cost of the test is around $300, and of course, requires supplying a blood sample taken by a health professional.

---

you can do to save your brain. There's compelling evidence, he says, that reducing calories can help stem everyday damage to neurons that over the years compromise normal aging brains, as well as brains afflicted with neurodegenerative disease.

Calories Make Old Brains

It's an indisputable tenet of aging, proved over and over in laboratory animals, that eating less food extends life spans. In short, calorie restriction slows down the aging process throughout your body, including your brain. A brain fed overgenerous amounts of calories gets older and damaged faster. When lab animals are put on low-calorie diets, trimming 30 to 40 percent off their food intake, they live one-third to one-half longer than expected. Such animals are usually only half the biological age of normally fed animals of the same chronological age. Everything about them is younger, including their brains and memories.

One reason is simply a matter of processing calories. In order to metabolize calories, you must burn oxygen, generating free radicals. Thus, the more calories consumed, the more free radicals created to damage cells including neurons. Consequently, the faster your mental faculties fade. Animals that burn fewer calories over a lifetime show much less free radical damage in their cells when they are examined after death. Besides curtailing free radical production, underfeeding also dramatically raises production of internal antioxidant defenses, supplying more brain-protective superoxide dismutase and glutathione to zap the free radicals that would destroy your neurons.

One bit of human confirmation: The islanders on Japanese Okinawa who for years ate a diet with 17 to 40 percent fewer calories than other Japanese had 30 to 40 percent less chronic disease, including neurodegenerative disorders such as Alzheimer's.

Cutting Calories Builds Stronger Brains

On a slightly different track, Dr. Mattson finds that restricting calories may help immunize brain cells against damage and disease in a different manner. He and colleagues have detected specific molecular changes in the brain cells of animals eating lower calorie diets. Remarkably, he finds that overeating weakens or primes brain cells for damage and conversely that restricting calories bucks up nerve cells, making them stronger and more resistant to damage. Underfed animals are much less apt to develop the signs of neuronal damage characteristic of degenerative brain diseases, such as Alzheimer's, Parkinson's, and Huntington's diseases.

In recent tests, Dr. Mattson cut the calorie intake of young rats (age two months—comparable to five years in humans) by 30 percent compared with rats allowed to eat as much as they wanted. All the rats were then subjected to brain toxins that mimic the destruction of neurons in the hippocampus, as inflicted by Alzheimer's, and destruction of nerve cells in the striatum, a brain region affected in Parkinson's. Afterward, the animals were taught to perform feats of memory, learning, and motor coordination. Unquestionably, the calorie-restricted animals performed much better on the tests of mental and motor functioning. "The beneficial effects of the dietary restriction were striking," said Dr. Mattson.

For example, rats free to eat anything showed severe memory deficits, but calorie-restricted rats exhibited little or no memory loss, despite the toxic assaults on their brains. In tests of balance and motor skills, calorie-restricted rats lasted three minutes before falling off a slowly rotating rod. Well-fed rats toppled off within a minute. But the proof of protection was seen when the animals' brain cells were meticulously examined postmortem. After three months, the well-fed rats had only half as many brain cells left as the calorie-restricted animals! The lower calorie intake had somehow shielded their brains from massive destruction.

The implications, of course, are that human brains could benefit as well. Indeed, new evidence suggests it's true. About ten years ago, Richard Mayeux, M.D., at Columbia University College of Surgeons and Physicians, started tracking 1500 healthy people to determine the impact of their diet on developing degenerative brain diseases. He has discovered that calorie intake does make a big difference. "After considering body size, people who took in fewer calories had a substantial reduction in the risk of Alzheimer's disease," he says. Moreover, the most "protected" brains belonged to the lower-calorie group who also ate a low-fat, high protein, high carbohydrate diet. Fewer calories also cut the risk of Parkinson's, he says.

Dr. Mattson says the "mild starvation" of fewer calories put stress on the brain cells causing them to grow stronger. "It's much like, the more you use your muscles, the stronger they become, and resistant to injury. It's also true for neurons," he says. Mattson theorizes that when stressed, the nerve cells "switch on" certain genes that increases levels of growth factor in the brain, making the cells more resistant to damage from free radicals, involved in brain degeneration.

It took a month or two of calorie restriction in rats before brain protection kicked in, says Dr. Mattson. That would be several years in humans. To meet the same calorie restrictions as the animals, typical Americans would have to shave off seven hundred to a thousand daily calories, bringing consumption down from an average 2500 to 3000 daily calories to 1800 to 2000 calories per day. Mattson, who is five feet nine inches and weighs 125 pounds, says he eats about 2000 to 2200 calories a day.

Cutting drastically down on calories is a hard sell to Americans, Dr. Mattson agrees. But he believes it's worth it considering the high stakes—your brain. He and other scientists are also looking for shortcuts, such as drugs or other less severe measures, that may do much the same thing as calorie restriction without the hardship. Still, even if you don't make severe reductions, curtailment to any degree may help ward off eventual mental decline. Every calorie not eaten and not burned means fewer free radicals to attack your brain cells.

BOTTOM LINE: *Burning more calories weakens brain cells and accelerates the aging of the brain.*

Caffeine: Everybody's Brain Fix?

Undeniably, we are a nation of caffeine junkies and the psychoactive drug profoundly affects our brains. At least 80 percent of adults in Western countries regularly consume caffeine in amounts large enough to affect brain functioning, say experts. And that doesn't count the millions of children who are hooked on caffeine-spiked colas and other soft drinks.

The major question: Is caffeine good or bad for the brain? It all depends on how your brain reacts to caffeine. Most people feel more cheerful and alert, more clear-headed and focused, more energetic and productive, even euphoric, after a dose of caffeine, say experts. Others become jittery, anxious, headachy, even at risk of panic attacks after drinking coffee or taking caffeine. It's mostly a matter of inherited biological individuality. It is also true that most people who use caffeine regularly tend to get mildly addicted, including children. In a small way caffeine has some of the qualities of "upper" drugs without the profound hazards, say some experts.

"There's no question caffeine is a mild psychomotor stimulant that produces effects qualitatively similar to very low doses of cocaine and amphetamine, provid-

ing classic stimulation—feelings of increased energy, well being, decreased sleepiness, talkativeness, more sociability and better ability to concentrate." —Roland Griffiths, Ph.D., leading caffeine researcher, Johns Hopkins University School of Medicine

Why Caffeine Gives Your Brain a Jolt

Surprisingly, caffeine is not a typical stimulant; it does not prod brain cells to perk up, hop to, become alert, and perform better. Caffeine, rather, works in a roundabout way. Instead of triggering release of "up" chemicals, it blocks the action of the neurotransmitter adenosine that ordinarily tells the brain to quiet down and go to sleep. Since the caffeine molecule chemically resembles adenosine, it can plop down on brain cell receptor sites, displacing adenosine. This prevents adenosine from stifling the enthusiasm of "upper" neurotransmitters, such as dopamine. Thus, caffeine, masquerading as adenosine, fools brain cells into remaining in a persistent state of excitability. A little caffeine goes a long way. Experts say that the caffeine in a couple of cups of coffee can knock out half the brain's adenosine receptors for a couple of hours, keeping your brain on high alert.

How Much of a Brain-Kick?

Even small amounts of caffeine increase alertness and concentration, relieve fatigue, and speed up reaction times. This was established by classic studies done at the Massachusetts Institute of Technology in the late 1980s by Harris R. Lieberman, Ph.D., and Richard Wurtman, M.D. In a group of men, they found that caffeine ranging from 32 milligrams in a carbonated cola to 256 milligrams in a ten-ounce mug of brewed coffee boosted performance on tests requiring alertness, concentration, and fast reactions. The conclusion: Even small amounts of caffeine are psychoactive, but the optimal dose appears to be 100 to 200 milligrams—one to two five-ounce cups of coffee—taken in the morning and again in late afternoon when caffeine wears off. Higher doses of caffeine did not rev up brain power further.

> **BOTTOM LINE:** *To boost brain performance, all you need is the caffeine in a cup of coffee in the morning and again at midday. Trying to further hype up your brain with more caffeine is usually futile and counterproductive.*

A Cup of Tea Does the Trick

Surprisingly, even drinking a single cup of tea, containing about 60 milligrams of caffeine—roughly half that of coffee—can give your brain an instant boost, speeding up reaction time and performance on mental tests. British researchers recently had subjects drink a cup of tea, or a cup of hot water spiked with 60 milligrams of caffeine, or the same beverages with no caffeine. Immediately afterward, investigators administered an 80-minute battery of mental performance tests. Amazingly, *within minutes of drinking the caffeine*, the subjects' reaction times speeded up, as evidenced by their quicker responses to the battery of tests. Their answers were also more accurate.

Indeed, drinking tea (or coffee) several times a day helps keep you alert and at higher mental performance levels, finds other recent British research. Drinking a cup of tea or coffee at 9 A.M., 2 P.M., and 7 P.M. preserved alertness and good cognitive performance throughout the day, which otherwise typically declines. When subjects drank only water during the day, their alertness and performance fell steadily. Also the beneficial impact on the brain was quick—evident within ten minutes. Further, researchers suspect the brain-boost was not entirely due to the caffeine alone, but to other biologically active ingredients in the tea or coffee.

Can Caffeine Boost Memory?

It's debatable, but there is some evidence that caffeine may sharpen memory. Researchers at London's National Addiction Centre tested 9003 adult caffeine users. Those who drank the most caffeine in coffee, and to a lesser extent in tea, performed best on a number of cognitive tests, including reaction time, verbal memory, and visual-spatial reasoning, than non-caffeine users. Older people got more of a mental boost from caffeine than younger people, concluded investigators.

Dutch researchers also found that caffeine can boost memory. Researchers at the University of Limburg in Maastricht had sixteen persons take a drug that impaired short-term and long-term memory. Consuming caffeine dramatically reversed the drug-induced impairment. Subjects who drank two to three small cups of coffee (250 milligrams caffeine) retrieved information from their long-term memory and recalled words from short-term and long-term memory tests normally; their reading speed and visual searches also improved almost to the non-drug level. Researchers attributed the memory enhancement to a stimu-

---

THE BIG THREE CAFFEINE SOURCES

Coffee, brewed: About 20 milligrams of caffeine per ounce.
Tea: About 5 milligrams of caffeine per ounce.
Cola: About 4 milligrams of caffeine per ounce.

---

lation of "cholinergic activity," or increases in activity of the "memory" neurotransmitter acetylcholine, which happens, they say, when caffeine blocks adenosine.

Italian investigators also showed that caffeine improves memory consolidation in experimental animals, as shown by their enhanced ability to remember how to find their way through mazes. But caffeine improved memory through mechanisms other than by blocking adenosine, researchers concluded.

Another reason caffeine might boost memory: It causes a slight adrenaline rush that clears up fuzzy brains. Adrenaline also triggers a rise in blood sugar (glucose) which in turn prods increased release of the memory enhancing neurotransmitter, acetylcholine.

Dr. Richard Restak, of George Washington University and an authority on the brain, recommends the "judicious use of caffeine" to help older people compensate for the slowing down of brain functioning.

More Is Not Better

On one test, caffeine flunks. You can't count on massive amounts of caffeine to improve your ability to make complex managerial decisions, according to tests at Penn State University. Researchers had twenty-four highly paid managers who normally consumed four or more cups of coffee daily (400 to 1000 milligrams of caffeine) take a six-hour video-computerized test of scenarios designed to test their skill at making complex managerial decisions.

A week later, the managers were told to take an extra 400 milligrams a day of caffeine in capsules. Although this is a lot of caffeine (bringing everybody's intake up to eight to fourteen cups of coffee a day), it's not unusual for people under stress to consume that much, said researchers. The subjects were then put through another simulated video-computer test of their complex managerial skills to determine whether they did better or worse.

Interestingly, under the influence of excess caffeine, they were 20 percent speedier in making decisions. But their decisions were not necessarily better. Indeed, the managers' capacity to take advantage of specific opportunities, a good predictor of real-world managerial success, deteriorated on the excessive doses of caffeine—perhaps because the managers jumped to action without taking enough time to remember and consider information relevant to the decision. In general, though, the excess caffeine had no impact on most measures of managerial effectiveness, researchers concluded.

Is Caffeine an Antidepressant?

Unquestionably, many people say caffeine puts them in a better mood. "Caffeine produces elevations of feelings of well-being, sometimes euphoria," agrees Dr. Griffiths at Johns Hopkins. New research by Dr. Lieberman, now at the U.S. Army Research Institute of Environmental Medicine in Natick, Massachusetts, shows that modest doses of caffeine (64 to 256 milligrams daily) boosted mood, as determined by a series of mood-assessment tests, in subjects who were young and old, male and female.

Dr. Lieberman suggests that caffeine has "an antidepressant-like" action. Backing up his finding, a couple of recent large scale population studies have tied coffee drinking to a lower risk of suicide.

"It seems not only possible, but likely, that some of the millions of heavy coffee drinkers are, in fact, using caffeine—consciously or not—to medicate themselves for depression, our most widespread psychiatric condition." —Melvin Konner, M.D., Emory University

Note: Some experts also observe that caffeine can *cause* depression in some persons and that getting off caffeine entirely *relieves* their depression.

Grumpy Without the Fix

Decidedly, research proves what most people know—that being deprived of your morning cup of coffee can make you irritable. In blind tests, Dr. Andrew Baum, professor of medical psychology at the Uniformed Services University of the Health Sciences in Bethesda, Maryland, set out cups of morning coffee with and without caffeine. It was easy to tell who got what even without the secret code. Subjects who unknowingly got the coffee or tea without caffeine were grumpy, lethargic, headachy, and performed poorly on mental tasks. On days they got the coffee with caffeine their mood soared; they were less stressed and did better on mental tests.

Although such dependence on caffeine may be distressing, Dr. Baum marveled that you need not constantly increase your caffeine intake to satisfy your cravings and get your morning fix, as you do with most addictive substances. Caffeine is unique, he said, in that a single cup gives your brain the same morning "jump-start" and mood-lift day after day, even if you are a heavy-duty caffeine consumer. There is no demand to raise the caffeine ante to satisfy your habit.

That's the good news. The bad news, of increasing concern to some scientists, is that caffeine is addictive; you can become dependent on it, and if you don't get your regular fix, you feel lousy. Some say that's the primary reason caffeine is so popular: Once hooked, you need it to alleviate the withdrawal symptoms of headaches, depression, and fatigue. Some even argue that much of caffeine's reputed boost of mental performance and mood may not be a real effect, but actually a "relief of withdrawal symptoms" in those already caffeine-addicted. That implies that caffeine primarily or solely improves performance and mood by erasing the need for a caffeine fix.

Hopkins's Dr. Griffiths says the effect of caffeine goes beyond correcting caffeine withdrawal. For example, British psychologist David M. Warburton, of the University of Reading, found that men ages eighteen to thirty who were not suffering caffeine deprivation or withdrawal improved in cognitive functions and mood when given 75 to 150 milligrams of caffeine—between half-a-cup and a cup and a-half-of-coffee. They scored higher on computerized tests of attention, problem solving, and delayed recall. The caffeine also lifted their moods, as measured by standard tests, making them more "clear-headed, happy, calm and less tense." Dr. Warburton concludes that caffeine works its magic, boosting absolute performance and mood, and not merely alleviating withdrawal symptoms of habituated users.

The Addiction Phenomenon

It's easy to become dependent on caffeine. Dr. Roland Griffiths recently found that more than half of a group of subjects suffered withdrawal symptoms after giving up the caffeine in a single daily cup of strong brewed coffee or three cans of caffeinated drink! They complained of headache, fatigue, lethargy, mood changes, muscle pain, stiffness, flu like feelings, nausea, and craving for caffeine.

In extreme cases, people deprived of caffeine become "functionally impaired in normal daily activities," finds Dr. Griffiths, "literally crippled by abstinence from caffeine."

Interestingly, other research shows that some heavy caffeine users—used to drinking ten cups a day—who quit caffeine do not suffer any significant withdrawal consequences.

Kids Are Addicted, Too

Perhaps even more worrisome: The same punishing withdrawal happens to a child deprived of regular fixes of caffeine. Because of the increased consumption of soft drinks, even bottled water with caffeine, as well as chocolate, youngsters are prime candidates for caffeine withdrawal. In one study, University of Minnesota researchers gave children, ages eight to twelve, 120 to 145 milligrams of caffeine a day (the amount in three to five caffeine-containing soft drinks) for about two weeks. When the caffeine was abruptly dis-

---

WHAT TO EXPECT IF YOU QUIT

Typical caffeine withdrawal symptoms: Headaches, primarily. Also depression, lethargy, irritability, muscle tension; in rare cases, nausea and vomiting.

How long will it last? A few days, maybe a week. Headaches usually begin in 12 to 24 hours after quitting caffeine.

How to avoid or lessen it? Don't stop caffeine cold turkey. Gradually decrease the intake of caffeine. A couple of ways: Reduce your coffee intake by a cup each day. Combine regular and decaf coffee, gradually increasing amounts of decaf until it is 100 percent. Even 25 milligrams of caffeine per day—in an ounce-and-a-half of brewed coffee—can ward off withdrawal headaches.

How much do you need to consume to become "dependent" or addicted to caffeine? As little as a morning cup of coffee or three to five colas a day can do the trick, leading to negative repercussions on your brain if you stop.

COLAS COUNT

You may not think that cola has the same caffeine-impact on the brain as coffee. It's a common misconception, but it's a myth, according to tests by psychiatrists at the University of Vermont. They found that caffeine consumed in either cola or coffee reaches peak levels in your saliva, and presumably your brain, at the same time. However, it is true that the amount of caffeine in a cola is one-third to one-half that of a regular cup of coffee. But even as little as the caffeine in four to six ounces of a cola has increased alertness.

continued, the kids had definite deterioration of brain function, lasting a couple of weeks. Within twenty-four hours of stopping caffeine, the children had slower reaction times and lower performance in a task requiring sustained attention.

Be aware, too, that caffeine can trigger even more serious neurological symptoms in children. If your child has a facial tic, a muscle spasm of the facial muscles, check his or her consumption of caffeine. Researchers at the University of Kansas Medical Center found that tics tended to appear when a child consumed caffeine and to disappear when the caffeine consumption stopped. Researchers concluded that caffeine may cause tics in susceptible children.

CAFFEINE ALERT! Many weekend headaches are probably a withdrawal symptom due to a lack of the usual workday quota of caffeine.

Caffeine's High Anxiety

Some brains are extremely sensitive to caffeine. In fact, caffeine-induced anxiety is far more common than realized. One study showed that 30 percent of adult users reported anxiety due to caffeine. As little as 250 milligrams a day—only two-and-a-half cups of coffee—can trigger anxiety in ordinary people. Much less may can trigger or aggravate anxiety and panic attacks in those particularly vulnerable to the disorder. Research at the National Institute of Mental Health even found that a dose of 750 milligrams (seven to eight 5-ounce cups of coffee) a day induced panic attacks in two of eight *normal* subjects with no history of panic disorder. Recent British studies show that caffeine worsens social anxiety.

Moreover, in susceptible individuals, only five or six cups of coffee a day can produce so-called "caffeine intoxication," a psychiatric disorder characterized by nervousness, excitement, restlessness, tachycardia (irregular heartbeats), insomnia, psychomotor agitation, and rambling thought and speech. Some people's brains are simply unable to tolerate caffeine.

> *"Some people may really need drugs to alleviate anxiety, but for an undetermined number of others, subtracting one drug—caffeine—may be of greater benefit than adding another."* —John F. Greden, M.D., formerly of Walter Reed Army Medical Center

How your brain reacts to caffeine may be inherited. One recent study suggests that heredity may account for one-third to one-half of your tolerance for caffeine and whether you suffer withdrawal symptoms. Recent brain scans reveal that individuals who are intolerant to caffeine metabolize caffeine differently. A new study compared the brain scans of heavy caffeine users and those intolerant to caffeine. The caffeine-intolerant reacted with "moderate to marked anxiety" when given the caffeine in about five cups of coffee for a 120-pound person. Also, brain scans showed disturbances in the way they metabolized caffeine; production of a specific brain chemical increased and blood flow to certain regions of the brain decreased. Such biological signs may help explain how caffeine produces anxiety and psychological distress in some people, researchers said.

> *"Caffeine, the most widely used behaviorally active drug in the world, produces very different reactions in different individuals."* —Larry Christensen, Ph.D., University of South Alabama

Caffeine and Sleep

Unfortunately, caffeine can put your brain on high alert, keeping you awake long after you want to go to sleep. It's no myth that caffeine is linked to chronic insomnia. If you're like most people, drinking a strong cup of coffee an hour before going to bed will disturb your sleep. In one Japanese study, subjects who consumed 150 milligrams of caffeine took an average 126 minutes to get to sleep, compared with 29 minutes for those who did not take caffeine. The caffeine-takers slept a total of about four-and-a-half hours; the non-caffeine drinkers, seven-and-a-half hours. Electrical recordings of the brain revealed that caffeine caused disruptions in normal sleep patterns and quality of sleep. Caffeine users tend to toss and turn more and wake up more during the night.

Since sleep deprivation is shown to actually damage brain cells, caffeine late in the day is not a good idea.

Best advice: Don't drink caffeine after late afternoon if you want a good night's sleep.

Note: It is also true that some people can drink caffeine and never have a sleep problem. Their brains are not as responsive to caffeine as other brains.

> **BRAIN ALERT:** If you are nursing an infant, it's a good idea not to consume caffeine; it ends up in the milk and ultimately in the infant's brain, where it has the same effect as on yours: Mainly, it could keep the baby awake and alert.

Caffeine and Blood Pressure

The prevailing wisdom is that caffeine raises blood pressure only temporarily and that the body adapts to the caffeine; thus, it is not a threat for people with high blood pressure over the long term. Some experts, including psychiatrist Dr. James D. Lane at Duke University Medical Center, disagree. Dr. Lane says his studies show that regular use of caffeine can keep blood pressure elevated, increasing normal blood pressure by ten or so points, enough to push a person over the edge into a high blood pressure category.

The rise appears greater in older people with high blood pressure, according to other research. A study at the West Australian Heart Research Institute in Perth showed that systolic blood pressure was nearly 5 points higher and diastolic pressure 3 points higher in older coffee drinkers (300 milligrams caffeine per day or 5 small cups of coffee) than in non-coffee-drinkers.

Dr. Lane firmly believes caffeine is an overlooked contributor to high blood pressure. His advice for those with high blood pressure: Gradually give up caffeine for a few weeks and see if blood pressure declines.

WHERE YOU GET CAFFEINE: MAJOR SOURCES

	Milligrams
Coffee:	
Brewed, 8 ounces	135
Instant, 8 ounces	95
Starbucks espresso, 1 ounce	89
Decaffeinated coffee, 8 ounces	.5
Tea:	
Lipton tea, 8 ounces	35–40
Snapple ice tea, all varieties, 16-ounce bottle	48
Herbal tea, all varieties	0
Soda: 12 ounces	
Jolt	71
Josta	58
Mountain Dew	55
Diet Coke	47
Coca-Cola	45
Dr. Pepper	41
Sunkist Orange Soda	40
Pepsi-Cola	37
7-UP	0
Sprite	0
Caffeinated Waters: 16.9 ounces	
Java Water	125
Krank20	100
Aqua Blast	90
Water Joe	60–70
Aqua Java	50–60
Ice Cream: 1 cup	
Ben & Jerry's No Fat Coffee	85
Starbucks Coffee Ice Cream	40–60
Häagen-Dazs Coffee	30
Yogurt: 8 ounces	

Dannon Coffee Yogurt	45
Stonyfield Farm Cappuccino	0
Chocolate: Hershey's Special Dark bar: 1.5 oz	31
Hershey Bar (milk chocolate): 1.5 ounces	10
Hot chocolate: 8 ounces	5

Source: The Center for Science in the Public Interest based on data from the National Coffee Association, the National Soft Drink Association, the Tea Council of the USA, and information provided by food and beverage companies, and J.J. Barone, H.R. Roberts (1996) "Caffeine Consumption," *Food Chemistry and Toxicology*.

Caffeine as Brain-Buster

You should restrict caffeine if:

- You have negative reactions to caffeine, such as tension, jitters, anxiety, headaches, nervousness, shakiness, low moods, low energy.
- You have anxiety disorder or panic attacks. Caffeine can aggravate anxiety and precipitate panic attacks in susceptible persons.
- You have borderline high blood pressure. Caffeine may push you over into high blood pressure.
- You are a pregnant or lactating woman. It can be detrimental to the fetus and nursing child.

BOTTOM LINE: *As a way of perking up the brain and fighting fatigue, caffeine is a beneficial, relatively benign psychoactive drug devoid of major health hazards for most people. For others more sensitive to it, caffeine can be a kind of brain poison, promoting anxiety, depression, psychiatric illness. Caffeine withdrawal is also an often unrecognized cause of headaches, low energy and low moods, for both adults and children.*

PART 3

BRAIN SUPPLEMENTS: WHAT TO TAKE FOR A MIRACLE BRAIN

How Vitamins, Minerals, and Other Supplements Can Boost Your Brain to the Max

Whether you are young, old, or in between, taking vitamin-mineral supplements can improve brain function, possibly boost performance on IQ tests, improve mood and memory, and slash the chances of brain deterioration as you get older. Indeed, the evidence is so compelling that it seems incredible everyone is not taking vitamins, minerals, and antioxidants to keep their brains functioning at peak levels for a lifetime.

As Dr. Denham Harman, professor emeritus at the University of Nebraska, and others demonstrated in animals or humans as long ago as the 1950s, your brain, general health, and longevity are initially shaped long before you are born by the vitamins and antioxidants your mother ingests during pregnancy and even before conception. A string of studies, many done a decade ago and seemingly lost to public consciousness, have found that giving multivitamins and specific vitamin supplements to schoolchildren can dramatically increase IQ scores. Research among adults of all ages also finds that certain vitamin and mineral supplements improve mood, learning ability, memory, attention span, eye-hand coordination, and reaction times, even in people who show no overt signs of deficiency.

Further, mountains of stunning evidence have piled up in the last few years, documenting that middle-aged and older people can stave off intellectual deterioration and even retrieve mental faculties thought lost forever by taking vitamins, particularly antioxidant vitamins and B vitamins. In one remarkable finding, vitamin E equaled a potent pharmaceutical drug in treating the most dreaded brain disease of all—Alzheimer's. Vitamins also protect the brains of normal healthy people. A recent random survey of 880 elderly men and women by European researchers showed that those with high vitamin and antioxidant blood levels had stronger intellectual powers, less depression, and less risk of losing their brains to dementia.

Then why isn't everyone downing vitamin supplements to maximize mental functioning? Since vitamins and minerals are generally safe in required doses and relatively inexpensive compared with remedies needed to rectify the potential damage to society in health and educational costs of not taking vitamins, why isn't the practice more widespread and medically encouraged?

One reason is conventional nutrition still maintains that the brain is not impaired unless the body is in a state of classic malnutrition, induced only after serious and prolonged deficiencies. Such malnutrition, characterized by overt physical signs of wasting away and rock bottom blood levels of nutrients, is considered rare in Western countries.

However, more daring researchers argue that the brain is the target of *subtle* deficiencies that leave it secretly impoverished long before any physical signs of conventional malnutrition are noticeable. It's well known that a wide range of vitamins and minerals are linked to psychological functioning and that many such nutrients are missing in typical high-fat, highly processed diets. "What is adequate to prevent physical signs and symptoms of malnutrition may not be adequate to prevent impaired mental function," says researcher Steven J. Schoenthaler at California State University.

Even the tiniest deficiencies could cause subtle and undetected disruption in psychological functioning, contends David Benton, a world-renowned research psychologist at University College in Swansea, Wales. "Cognitive activity," says Dr. Benton, "involves the summated activity of many billions of neurones, and countless biochemical pathways and their associated enzymes. It may well be that relatively small dietary deficiences that are dismissed as causing only minor changes to the activity of a single enzyme, will along with many other similar minor effects, have a measurable and potentially important cumulative influence on cerebral functioning."

Much evidence, in fact, raises the specter that modern western society is rife with a pernicious form of "subclinical" (symptomless) or "marginal" malnutrition that leaves no obvious traces of brain malfunction. The brain may get enough vitamins and minerals to appear to function "normally." But is it really operating at *optimal* levels? Some researchers believe substantial segments of the population do not get nearly the levels of vitamins and minerals needed to optimize brain function. Deterioration in mental function previously attributed to "normal aging," may, in fact, be at least partly due to subtle undetected and correctable deficiencies of specific vitamins needed by the brain, says Katherine Tucker, associate professor of nutritional epidemiology at Tufts University. "It's a new and powerful idea," she says, "with accumulating evidence to support it."

It seems obvious that the poor-quality, high-fat, low-vitamin diets of many Americans, sadly, including school-children, are inadequate to fuel peak brain performance, and that undernourished brains might perk up when supplied vitamin and mineral supplements. In short, our brains quietly survive and endure on poor diets in a permanent state of lethargy that we accept as "normal" because we can't imagine otherwise. We are unaware that we have the potential to be smarter and feel better—that our brains, when properly nourished, can reach for and achieve more and function at higher levels.

BOTTOM LINE: *Vitamins, impressive studies show, can help ensure maximum brain functioning from birth to old age.*

Raise Your Child's IQ with Multivitamins

Wouldn't it be remarkable if taking vitamins could raise a child's IQ score? It may seem preposterous. That's what British psychologist David Benton, thought, too, until he decided to investigate. He is now convinced that giving vitamin-mineral supplements to children has the potential to significantly boost their scores on intelligence tests. The first evidence came from his 1988 double-blind study of twelve-year-old schoolchildren published in *The Lancet*, a prestigious British medical journal.

Dr. Benton gave thirty children a special vitamin-mineral supplement and thirty others a dummy pill or placebo for eight months. The kids took standard intelligence tests before and after. Scores on the so-called "verbal" part of the test did not change. But, remarkably, the scores of vitamin-takers on the "nonverbal" intelligence test soared an average nine points—up from 111 to 120, compared with a mere one point in non-supplemented kids.

Dr. Benton was surprised, but says it makes sense. No one would expect vitamins to raise *verbal* IQ scores because they measure achievement and reflect cultural, educational, and environmental factors, such as a better vocabulary, he says. "And, for sure, taking vitamins is not going to give you a better vocabulary." But tests of nonverbal intelligence are another matter. Nonverbal intelligence reflects basic biological functioning, or brain potential. You can't elevate it through education. For example, as brain weight increases in infants and young children, so do their scores on nonverbal intelligence tests, says Dr. Benton. It is logical then, he says, that vitamins would affect nonverbal, biologically influenced intelligence, but not learned verbal IQs.

Dr. Benton's report stirred up much public and scientific controversy in Great Britain, including a favorable BBC TV documentary and a court trial resulting in fines of a vitamin company that trumpeted the results to sell thousands of bottles of vitamins to worried parents. Some scientists rejected the proposition that vitamins could raise IQ. Others disagreed on what percentage of children might benefit. Dr. Benton argued that if there was a reasonable chance of boosting IQ, considering that vitamins are so inexpensive, it would be smart to take the supplements at least as "insurance."

Other research has backed up Dr. Benton's findings. One is a 1991 study by Steven J. Schoenthaler, a California State University criminologist long interested in a connection between diet and delinquent behavior. He gave twenty-six institutionalized juvenile delinquents, ages thirteen to sixteen, either a multivitamin-mineral supplement or a placebo for thirteen weeks. Before and after the supplementation, he tested their intelligence by the Wechsler Intelligence Scale for Children. He also assessed their brain function by a special computerized EEG machine, and measured their blood concentrations of ten vitamins and seven minerals to judge their nutritional status.

After thirteen weeks of vitamin-mineral supplements, the children's verbal scores on the IQ test did not change, as expected, but nonverbal IQ scores of the vitamin-takers went up an average six points. One youngster's IQ score skyrocketed 25 points—from 117 to an astonishing 142. Another's rose from 100 to 123. The improvement in scores led Dr. Schoenthaler to conclude that "underlying malnutrition may be a likely cause of academic difficulties." Also remarkable, a high incidence of EEG brain wave abnormalities virtually vanished in those getting vitamins. And there was a possible bonus: Antisocial behavior—such as violent attacks on staff and other residents in the facility—declined in those whose nutritional status improved, said Schoenthaler.

The idea got increasing support when prominent British nutritional authority John Yudkin at Kings College in London became intrigued and joined Dr. Schoenthaler in a study of 615 eighth and tenth grade children. After thirteen weeks, about 45 percent of those taking supplements with 100 percent of the RDA, gained 15 or more points in nonverbal IQ compared with 20 percent in the placebo group. Researchers concluded that "dietary supplementation improved fluid intelligence estimates by a minimum of 6 points, with an average of 11 points and a maximum of 21 points"—a substantial boost, suggesting that the brain is undermined by subtle hidden vitamin deficiencies easily corrected by supplements.

Another 1991 study by Dr. Benton and Richard Cook in Swansea, Wales, showed that multivitamin-mineral supplements raised intelligence scores of six-year-old children over eight points, compared with a placebo. The rise was attributed to the youngsters' increased ability to concentrate.

In an interview in 1998, Dr. Benton said at least seven studies consistently show that vitamin supplements can cause "a relatively large" increase in youngsters' nonverbal intelligence scores. In fact, Dr. Benton asserts that, based on research, from one-third to one-half of all children might improve IQ scores by taking vitamins. That's an astounding 23 to 35 million children under age eighteen in the United States! "No known pharmacological drug can cause this kind of impact," he adds.

So what explains such a phenomenon? A particularly striking finding in these studies is that kids whose IQs shot up the most—or at all—also improved most in nutritional status. The supplements normalized blood levels of vitamins and minerals in youngsters who initially had abnormally low blood levels. This is the major clue to the stunning results, says Dr. Benton. He contends the vitamins work because they correct substandard intellectual functioning due to marginal deficiencies caused by a poor diet. Unquestionably, subclinical deficiencies of micronutrients disrupt psychological functioning, says Dr. Benton. Brain cells starving for nutrients cannot function optimally.

Proof comes from blood tests. Most children whose IQ scores rise also show a rise in blood levels of vitamins, indicating their bodies *needed* the vitamins. If you are well nourished, the body will not take up unneeded nutrients.

How can you know if your child lacks key nutrients and might improve intellectual performance by taking vitamins? You can't, because it depends not only on diet but on individual biochemistry. Everybody responds differently to vitamin supplementation, says Dr. Benton. His view: Taking vitamin supplements will not improve every child's IQ scores. But since it is impossible to determine who will benefit and many kids eat nutritionally substandard diets, the gamble seems well worth it—especially since vitamins are relatively inexpensive and are beneficial throughout the body. It's a bet with no downside and the benefits could be phenomenal, not only to individual children but to society as a whole. As Dr. Benton says, in profound understatement, "It's good insurance." And who wouldn't want to take out insurance on their child's brains?

> *"Our studies show, we believe conclusively, that adding vitamins and minerals to the diets of children who have no obvious physical signs of nutrient deficiency can nevertheless produce an increase in their IQ scores."*
> —John Yudkin, emeritus professor of nutrition at King's College, London

What's in the IQ-Boosting Pills?

There is no unusual magic in the particular vitamin-mineral formulas shown to boost childhood performance on IQ tests. The supplements generally contain moderate amounts of a wide range of basic vitamins and minerals typical of many multi-vitamin combinations. For example Dr. Benton's original formula that dramatically boosted nonverbal IQ scores included 100 micrograms of folic acid, 12 milligrams of B_6, 50 milligrams of niacin, 50 milligrams of pantothenic acid, 4 milligrams of thiamin, 5 milligrams of riboflavin, 500 milligrams of vitamin C, 70 IU of vitamin E, 200 micrograms of chromium, 7 milligrams of magnesium, 1.3 milligrams of iron, 10 milligrams of zinc, 70 milligrams of choline, plus 50 milligrams of bioflavonoids. Such doses are considered sufficient to correct most deficiencies.

Best Advice: Any good-quality daily supplement with 100 percent of the recommended daily doses of a variety of vitamins and minerals is likely to provide the desired "insurance" to help guarantee that your child's brain is sufficiently nourished to function optimally.

Note: Even if your child scores better on IQ tests after taking vitamin supplements, don't expect major changes in scholastic performance. What has improved is the child's intellectual "potential," says Dr. Benton. Improved intellectual "performance" requires more, including individual effort and intellectual stimulation, and is likely to come gradually. "Any benefits are likely to be subtle and long-term rather than dramatic," says Dr. Benton.

> **BOTTOM LINE:** *Taking vitamin supplements does not push a kid's brain beyond normal capacity. A lack of the vitamins causes a youngster to perform below capacity. Or in Dr. Benton's words: "It's not that vitamins increase intelligence. It's that a poor diet lowers performance on intelligence tests."*

MULTIVITAMINS BOOST ADULT BRAINS

Can multivitamins also stimulate increased brain function in fully mature adult brains, even those that appear to be well nourished? There's good evidence for it. Many adults, too, have marginal subclinical deficiencies of vitamins that can be corrected by taking vitamins, stimulating better brain function. Further, vitamins in excess of the so-called recommended daily allowances could also have a kind of pharmacological effect—creating supranormal advantages to the brain above what would be expected from normal nutrition.

In one double-blind test, Dr. Benton had 127 healthy

"I OWE IT ALL TO VITAMINS"
—DAME BARBARA

British romance author Dame Barbara Cartland, in a 1992 letter to the *Guardian* newspaper, credited vitamins for her long and prodigious writing career. "I am 91," she wrote, "and I have just broken the record [*Guinness Book* of Records] by writing more books than any other English author—570. . . . I have also achieved the world record by writing for 17 years an average of 23 books. I would not have done this without vitamins. All my children and grandchildren have taken them. My eldest grandson passed the difficult examinations for chartered accountancy with honours. My second grandson won the debating cup at the Bar and my third passed so highly into Oxford that they offered him any college of his choice. They all say they owed this to the vitamins I gave them."

adults, men and women ages seventeen to twenty-seven, take either a placebo or a multivitamin supplement of nine vitamins for an entire year. It included moderately high doses of vitamin A, thiamin, riboflavin, vitamin B_6, vitamin B_{12}, vitamin C, vitamin E, folic acid, biotin, and nicotinamide. All subjects were given a battery of computer generated psychometric tests (to measure reaction time, intelligence, and so forth) before supplementation and every three months after supplementation.

Surprisingly, the vitamins had the greatest benefits on the mental functioning of females. Generally, women vitamin-takers had faster reaction times and processed information more quickly. *In all cases, when vitamin status improved, so did cognitive functioning in women.* Such improvement was most closely linked to improvements in vitamin B_6 status. Why women did better than men is unclear, but may be related to interactions between the B vitamins and estrogen, theorized researchers.

Want to Keep Your Brain Young? Take Vitamins

As more researchers unravel the mysteries of the aging brain, it's indisputable that older people with high blood levels of certain vitamins and antioxidants have better intellectual vitality. Exciting new evidence shows that there may be no better way to protect your brain from the ravages of so-called "normal aging," than by packing in vitamins, particularly B vitamins and antioxidants through diet and supplements. Blood levels of such nutrients may be an indicator of age-related memory and other mental abilities.

A team of researchers at the University of New Mexico, headed by James S. Goodwin, M.D., first brought that fact to medical attention in a 1983 issue of the *Journal of the American Medical Association*. The investigators suspected that "subclinical" or mild undetected vitamin deficiencies might be linked to subtle cognitive impairment in normal healthy independent-living older Americans. They studied 260 men and women ranging from ages sixty to ninety-four years old in the Albuquerque area. Remarkably, none took any prescription medications or had any diagnosed serious medical problems that could affect nutritional or cognitive status. The subjects appeared in excellent health.

All were given standardized tests of memory, abstract thinking, and problem solving abilities designed to detect minimal changes in mental status.

Here's what they found: Generally, the more vitamin C and various B vitamins in the blood, the better the mental function scores. The gap was particularly dramatic between those with the very lowest and highest vitamin blood levels. For example, those in the top 90 percentiles of blood vitamin C made about 20 percent fewer errors on the reasoning and problem-solving tests and scored nearly 25 percent better in the memory tests than those in the bottom 10 percentiles for vitamin C. Those with lower B_{12} also did worse on both memory and reasoning tests; those with low riboflavin or folic acid did worse on abstract calculating abilities. Thus, the research suggests that you increase your chances of good mental function as you age by maintaining high blood levels of B vitamins and vitamin C.

When Asenath La Rue, and colleagues at the University of New Mexico, restudied the above group six years later, they found essentially the same thing: High vitamin blood levels predicted high cognitive test scores. They also found that those taking supplements consistently had a "higher cognitive performance" than non-supplement-takers. Notably, those taking B vitamins scored better on memory performance and abstract thinking tests. Of high interest, many of the vitamin-taking subjects (ages sixty-six to ninety) "scored as well or better than younger adults on verbal memory," researchers concluded.

When researchers at the University of Hawaii recently tested the cognitive functioning of 3735 Japanese-American elderly men who were part of the long-term Honolulu Heart Program, they found that those who scored best were taking vitamins or had taken them for the previous four years. Regardless of age, education, or history of stroke, those currently taking multivitamins or vitamin C or vitamin E separately had the best intellectual function. There was a particularly strong protective effect for those who had taken vitamin C and vitamin E for the previous four years. Researchers suggest that the antioxidant activity of the vitamins retarded age-related cognitive decline.

Similarly, German researchers have found that a vitamin deficiency has cruel consequences for the functioning of older brains, including memory and mood. In 1986, investigators at the University of Gottingen and the University of Giessen compared the vitamin blood status of a group of sixty older men and women (ages sixty-five to ninety-one) and their scores on a variety of mental tests. Those who had substandard levels of any vitamin, especially thiamin, riboflavin, vitamin B_{12}, and vitamin C, were much more apt to be emotionally unstable, depressed, excitable, nervous, anxious, angry, irritable, easily discouraged, and fatigued. For example, those with low vitamin status were two-and-a-half times more apt to be fatigued and angry and twice as likely to be excitable and irritable. Those who lacked vitamins also had poorer short-term memories and slower reactions times. The researchers concluded that "behavior impairments, traceable by psychometric tests, seem most frequently to be the earliest clinical signs of vitamin deficiency."

Virtually every day exciting new research shows that various supplements encourages optimal brain functioning. Here's the latest evidence of the brain-boosting power of the B vitamins, vitamin E, vitamin C, coenzyme Q10, lipoic acid, ginkgo, phosphatidlyserine, and several other promising supplements for the brain.

Folic Acid
Revitalizes Memory

It's scientifically indisputable that your brain cannot function at peak form if you are low in the B vitamin folic acid. Extensive research shows that a deficit of folic acid is a common, but often hidden, culprit in various minor and severe psychiatric problems, as well as strokes. If you are depressed, you may lack folic acid. If your carotid (neck) arteries, which carry blood and oxygen to your brain, clog up, a major reason could be a folic acid deficiency. Folic acid is also abnormally low in people with dementia and Alzheimer's disease. Even perfectly healthy older people who lack folic acid score lower on tests of cognitive function, including memory.

More than twenty-five studies done between 1966 and 1990 show that psychiatric patients tend to be deficient in folic acid. In one study, fully 100 percent of older people diagnosed with vascular dementia and acute confusional state were deficient in folic acid. In other studies, 50 percent of those hospitalized with depression and 36 percent with schizophrenia had low blood levels of folic acid. This is compared with so-called healthy "control" subjects of whom only 3 to 8 percent showed folic acid deficiency.

BRAIN ALERT: *Blood tests typically find that from one-fifth to one-half of people with psychiatric complaints have low folic acid! The figure soars to 80 to 90 percent in older people with psychological disorders.*

MAJOR GLITCHES, MINOR GLITCHES

Skimping on folic acid also affects the brains of young people, and can produce subtle changes in mood and memory at all ages that are usually dismissed as just part of life's ordinary ups and downs. German researchers at the University of Giessen discovered that young men who ate diets low in folic acid suffered poor emotional stability, poor concentration, unusual introversion, a lack of self-confidence, and low mood. Eight weeks of moderate doses of folic acid, found in multivitamin pills, brought dramatic improvement.

In one famous test, a scientist deliberately ate a folic acid-deficient diet for three months. He suffered sleeplessness, forgetfulness, and irritability. Amazingly, his symptoms vanished within two days after he started taking folic acid supplements.

Many people may have what Canadian researcher M.I. Botez at the University of Montreal describes as a "folic-acid-deficiency syndrome," characterized by fatigue, mild or moderate depression, minor neurological signs, and gastrointestinal disorders. When Dr. Botez gave a very high pharmacological daily dose of 15 milligrams of folic acid to 50 sufferers, their verbal performance and IQ scores improved. Fully 85 percent declared their mood improvement as "very good" or "good."

In other studies schizophrenia patients have improved after taking folic acid. In a large, multicenter study of elderly depressed patients with mild to moderate dementia, Italian researchers achieved spectacular results with very high doses of methylfolate (a form of folic acid). It proved to be as effective in relieving symptoms of depression as the antidepressant drug trazodone. Among psychiatric patients, those receiving methylfolate were released from the hospital earlier, had less depression and better social functioning than those with low folic acid levels.

Although many people are still unaware of the psychiatric benefits of folic acid, the medical evidence leaves no doubt the vitamin is linked to minor mental glitches as well as serious depression, dementia, memory loss, schizophrenia, stroke and even autism and attention deficit disorder in children.

BRAIN ALERT: *A scarcity of folic acid is perhaps our most serious and widespread vitamin deficiency.*
- *About 60 percent of middle-aged men are deficient in folic acid.*
- *The average American over age fifty takes in a mere 235 micrograms of folic acid daily.*
- *Almost 90 percent of Americans consume less than the 400 micrograms of folic acid daily needed to curb the brain toxin homocysteine.*

DEPRESSED? THINK FOLIC ACID

Depression is the brain's most common reaction to low folic acid. Dozens of reports link depression with low folic acid, according to Harvard professors Jonathan E. Alpert, M.D., and Maurizio Fava, M.D. In fact, they say depression is the most common neuropsychiatric sign of a folic acid deficiency. From 15 to 38 percent of adults diagnosed with depression have borderline low or deficient blood levels of folic acid. Low folic acid, surprisingly, is a better indicator of depression than low vitamin B_{12}. Usually, the greater the folic acid deficit, the more severe the depression and the longer it lasts. One study of 44 people noted that even low-normal levels of folic acid predicted longer episodes of depression.

Another problem: If you're taking antidepressant drugs, they don't work as well if you are low in folic acid. This helps explain why some depressed persons are resistant to antidepressant drug therapy. Bringing folic acid up to par often helps relieve depression and makes standard antidepressants work better, concluded Drs. Alpert and Fava.

Adding even tiny amounts of folic acid can make a remarkable difference. In one double-blind study of seventy-five manic-depression patients on the drug lithium, only 200 micrograms of folic acid—the amount in three-quarters of a cup of cooked spinach—taken for a year dramatically elevated efficacy of the drug in reducing occurrence and duration of depression symptoms. And folic acid alone often brings astounding success. When Harvard's Dr. Fava gave twenty elderly depressed patients a large pharmacological dose of folic acid for six weeks, alone without any other drug whatsoever, a whopping 81 percent of them got better.

It's not totally clear how folic acid alleviates depression, but expert Dr. Simon Young at McGill University in Canada, says it's known that folic acid deficiency depresses production of the brain's natural antidepressant, serotonin. Sufficient folic acid, as expected, raises serotonin, relieving depression.

FOLIC ACID REVERSES MEMORY LOSS

As you age, folic acid becomes especially critical. Older brains are particularly vulnerable to harm from low folic acid. In 1997 a team of Italian researchers headed by M. Fioravanti, Department of Psychiatric Science and Psychological Medicine at the University of Rome, reviewed over forty international scientific papers on folic acid, cognition, and aging published in the previous ten years. They concluded that low folic acid levels, just like low B_{12} levels, in older people with intellectual decline may stem from an intestinal problem in absorbing folic acid. Further, they confirmed that folic acid supplements restored memory in aging brains.

In one double-blind study, the Italian investigators tested folic acid in thirty elderly patients with low blood folic acid and mild to moderate memory loss within the past two years. Half got a high pharmacological dose (15 milligrams) of folic acid daily for two months, the other half got a placebo. Decidedly, those getting folic acid scored higher on memory tests; their attention span also increased.

Most striking, the worse the initial folic acid deficiency, the greater the memory improvement. Also remarkable: Memory improved in a mere sixty days, indicating that folic acid may contribute to an amazingly quick fix, considering memory had been on the downslide for two years.

This study, along with new research from Tufts University, suggests that numerous older people suffer from an undetected "subclinical" folic acid deficiency, despite the appearance of good nutrition, that harms their memory and robs them of their minds. Folic acid shortage is, of course, not the total explanation for age-related memory loss, but it is a hidden cause of some magnitude, which is all the more needless since it is so easily corrected by supplements. Don't overlook folic acid deficiency as a thief of memory.

FOLIC ACID VS. STROKES

The big news is that folic acid helps protect aging brains from destructive vascular events, such as mini and major strokes as well as something called "white matter intensities"—brain abnormalities linked to cognitive decline. These smaller corrosions of the brain that go unnoticed are "really a much bigger problem than anyone has recognized," says Tufts researcher Dr. Tucker. Enter folic acid as savior.

Scientists now say that a blood factor called homocysteine, an amino acid, is a major villain in mental decline, vascular dementia, and strokes. They also know that the best cure for high homocysteine is folic acid. In the absence of sufficient folic acid, this toxic homocysteine piles up wildly in the blood. The possible result: a narrowing and clogging of the carotid artery, as well as of the small cerebral blood vessels that carry oxygen and glucose to the brain. Vitamins B_6 and B_{12} also help suppress homocysteine, but folic acid is by far the most powerful. Thus, at least 400 micrograms of folic acid a day in a supplement is necessary to curtail homocysteine and cut your risk of stroke. (For more on the hazards of homocysteine to your brain, see page 307.)

FOLIC ACID WAVES OFF ALZHEIMER'S
High levels of folic acid may also help ward off the brain destruction in Alzheimer's disease, according to exciting new findings by David Snowdon, M.D., at the University of Kentucky. In a large ongoing study of brain degeneration in elderly nuns, Dr. Snowdon previously detected higher levels of lycopene (from tomatoes) in the blood of sisters who functioned better mentally and physically in old age. Now Dr. Snowdon has discovered that the most massive damage from Alzheimer's occurred in the brains of those with the lowest blood levels of folic acid. An examination of thirty brains revealed that the most severe atrophy and abnormal configuration of plagues and tangles typical of advanced Alzheimer's, strongly matched blood samples with the lowest concentrations of folic acid. The implication: That low folic acid predicts Alzheimer's and high folic

acid helps prevent it. How? The obvious possibility: by controlling homocysteine that otherwise may damage nerve cells directly or indirectly by provoking ministrokes and other injuries in cerebral vessels. It's also possible that folic acid has some other brain-protecting abilities unrelated to homocysteine.

BRAIN ALERT: *Only one in ten Americans gets the amount of folic acid needed to curb high homocysteine, according to Harvard researchers.*

How Much to Take?

Most experts say 400 micrograms of folic acid daily are sufficient to keep homocysteine in check. People with depression and memory problems may need more. Dr. Young suggests that a dose below 1,000 micrograms or 1 milligram per day is enough to bring the brain back into working order in most circumstances.

Caution: Folic acid supplements can interfere with anticonvulsant drugs, and may "mask" pernicious anemia. Be sure to take B_{12} along with folic acid.

BOTTOM LINE: *Folic acid is not a trivial brain nutrient. A lack can contribute to a range of brain disturbances from minor mood changes, such as irritability, to thinking problems, forgetfulness, severe depression, and dementia. A modest dose of 400 micrograms to a maximum of 1000 micrograms daily can generally erase concern. Don't take higher doses without medical supervision.*

Vitamin B$_6$
Boosts Memory

Failing to get enough vitamin B$_6$ can bring psychological distress and suboptimal brain performance. You are likely to be more irritable, depressed, angry, fatigued, confused, less able to concentrate, and your memory may suffer, according to recent research. No question, vitamin B$_6$ can have a profound effect on neurological functioning. For one reason, the vitamin is needed to synthesize neurotransmitters, including serotonin, dopamine, norepinephrine, GABA, and taurine. Research suggests that a lack of B$_6$, in particular, leads to lower serotonin levels in the brain, and to consequent drops in mood, possibly even severe depression. In animals B$_6$ deficiencies are tied to central nervous system damage.

MEMORY LOSS ANTIDOTE
Although B$_6$ is important for good mental functioning at all ages, you especially need it to keep memory intact as you get older. Dutch psychologists in a double-blind controlled study have found that giving only 20 milligrams of B$_6$ daily to healthy men ages seventy to seventy-nine for three months slightly improved their long-term memory. Specifically, the takers of B$_6$ were better able to transfer newly learned verbal information into their long-term memory. Further, there was a direct correlation between a rise in B$_6$ blood status and increased memory function. The conclusion: Taking vitamin B$_6$ may reduce age-related memory decline. However, the researchers also noted that

extremely high blood levels of B_6 may impair memory, so doses should be moderate, not excessive.

Echoing the impact of B_6 on memory is Tufts University research by Katherine Tucker that links high B_6 blood levels with better memory among seventy middle-aged and elderly men. Men with high B_6 were dramatically better in recalling sequenced lists of numbers, words, and matched items. In a test of so-called "working memory"—the simultaneous storage and processing of new information—men with the highest blood B_6 scored 30 percent higher in recalling numbers backwards, regardless of age. They also recalled the most items. In a larger follow-up study, Tufts researchers found that older men with high B_6 also had better "delayed recall"—the ability to recall the details of a story read to them.

Interestingly, Tufts investigators found B_6 a stronger memory booster in middle-aged men than in older men. On one memory test, middle-aged men highest in B_6 had double the scores of younger men with the lowest B_6. Indeed, B_6 status predicted memory success. The more B_6 in the blood, the better the men's memory, regardless of other factors, such as education. Also, the memory performance of those with the least B_6 was not abnormally low. It's just that the men with the high B_6 did much better.

Further, nearly one-half of the men in the study had low blood levels of B_6, suggesting widespread subtle deficits in memory that could be easily corrected.

How does B_6 boost memory? One way: by helping lower homocysteine, a factor in the blood, tied to various mental disturbances including intellectual decline and dementia. However, that is not the entire explanation, says Tufts Dr. Tucker. B_6 boosts memory, regardless of its control of homocysteine, she has found. "I don't think we know right now the exact mechanism by which B_6 helps regulate memory." She speculates it could have something to do with B_6's role in the metabolism of amino acids.

How much? B_6 can be tricky for the brain, since both deficiencies and excesses can produce neurological disturbances. Experts suggest from 10 to 50 milligrams of B_6 per day to help keep homocysteine levels down. As little as 300 to 500 milligrams daily of B_6 might cause neuropathy in some individuals, although most cases result from more than that. Considered a safe dose: no more than 200 milligrams per day.

Vitamin B$_{12}$
Prevents "Senility"

What you don't know about vitamin B$_{12}$ can literally take your mind away. Unfortunately, it's a well-kept secret that a deficiency of vitamin B$_{12}$, which is alarmingly common, can lead to neurological damage, including disorientation, memory problems, and dementia. A recent survey found that sixty percent of a group of older people diagnosed with B$_{12}$ deficiency had no idea that a shortage of the vitamin could be so devastating to the brain. "The lack of knowledge about vitamin B$_{12}$ deficiency is astounding," said Dr. Robert M. Schmidt, professor of preventive medicine at California Pacific Medical Center in San Francisco and a board member of the local American Society on Aging that conducted the survey.

The awful neurological consequences of a B$_{12}$ deficit typically sneak up, originating in midlife, but do not become noticeable until twenty or thirty years later in the sixties or seventies. "A vitamin B$_{12}$ deficiency develops very slowly over many years and oddly, often affects the brain and nervous system entirely and nothing else," according to the late John Lindenbaum, M.D., an authority on vitamin B$_{12}$ at New York's Columbia Presbyterian Medical Center. He noted that a B$_{12}$ deficiency is often not detected by conventional blood tests.

The cause is usually not a faulty diet. You can't count on foods high in B$_{12}$ to save you from a deficiency as you get older. The real culprit is a biological fact of life. As you age, you can lose your ability to absorb vitamin B$_{12}$ from food. This condition, called atrophic gastritis, means your stomach progressively secretes less hydrochloric acid, pepsin, and intrinsic factor—a protein needed to absorb B_{12} from food—than when you were younger.

Atrophic gastritis is startlingly common. It becomes more prevalent with each passing year after middle age, and affects up to half of all Americans over age sixty, according to one study. But since it takes the body so long to exhaust stores of B_{12}, deficiency symptoms can take years to appear. Yet, silently and without hints of trouble, the B_{12} you eat goes to waste and your nervous system eventually begins to feel and respond to B_{12} starvation. Gradually, lacking B_{12} nourishment, the outer layer of nerve fibers deteriorate, giving rise to neurologic abnormalities, including loss of balance, muscle weakness, incontinence, mood disturbances, dementia, and psychosis.

The signs of B_{12} deficiency are often described as "pseudo-senility" because they so closely mimic those of age-related intellectual decline. Numerous older people with failing memory and other unexplained mental disturbances have been diagnosed with irreversible "senility" or Alzheimer's when in fact the cause was a very reversible deficiency of vitamin B_{12}. A recent Israeli study found that up to 16 percent of older people with dementia actually had a B_{12} deficiency.

However, a lack of B_{12} may lead to full-blown Alzheimer's disease. A recent British study by David Smith at Oxford University found that older people with abnormally low blood levels of vitamin B_{12} were four times more apt to develop Alzheimer's disease. A probable reason: the link with homocysteine, a blood factor thought to damage blood vessels and have direct toxic effects on brain cells. B vitamins, including folic acid, B_6 and B_{12}, help suppress homocysteine. In the British study, those deficient in B_{12} also had the highest levels of dangerous homocysteine.

Keeping the lid on homocysteine also cuts your risk of "brain attack," or strokes. B vitamins can help keep carotid arteries, that feed the brain, from closing.

> **BRAIN ALERT:** *The average American woman over age fifty gets only 43 to 48 percent of the recommended dose of B_{12} in her diet. Men of the same age get 62 to 75 percent, according to the U.S. Department of Health and Human Services.*
>
> *Everyone over age fifty should take supplements of B_{12} to help prevent neurologic damage due to deficiencies caused by malabsorption or "atrophic gastritis."*
> —National Academy of Sciences

The important fact is the sooner you catch and correct a B_{12} deficiency, the greater the chances of full recovery. If the brain is deprived of B_{12} for long periods, brain damage can become permanent. Dr. Robert Russell, Tufts University warns: "Always suspect a vitamin B_{12} deficiency if an older person develops unexplained neuropsychiatric problems."

Better yet, don't wait for a brain-busting B_{12} deficiency to occur. Take B_{12} supplements as insurance. They may not totally prevent a deficiency, but they sharply cut your risk. A recent study of 400 older people found that 40 percent of those not taking a vitamin supplement had low B_{12} compared with only 12 percent of those taking a daily supplement containing on average a mere 6 micrograms of B_{12}. In other words, non-multivitamin-takers tripled their risk of B_{12} deficiency.

The B_{12} in supplements is a "crystalline" form which is much better absorbed than B_{12} in food, despite low levels of stomach acid due to atrophic gastritis. You can take B_{12}

HOW MUCH IS TOO MUCH FOR YOUR BRAIN?

High doses of vitamins and minerals could become toxic to the body and brain. Here is a guide to how much is safe:

After an extensive review of the medical research on vitamins and minerals, John Hathcock, Ph.D., formerly with the Food and Drug Administration, and now with the Council for Responsible Nutrition, compiled the following chart of supplement risks for adults:

Nutrient	Daily Safe Dose*	Lowest Dose Known to Cause Harm
Vitamin A (retinol)	10,000 IU	21,600 IU (liver damage)
Beta carotene	25 mg	none known
Vitamin D	800 IU	2000 IU
Vitamin E	1200 IU	none known
Vitamin C	Over 1,000	none known
Thiamin (B_1)	50 mg	none known
Riboflavin (B_2)	200 mg	none known
Niacin		
Nicotinic acid:	500 mg	1000 (500 mg slow release)
Nicotinamide:	1500 mg	3000 mg
Pyridoxine (B_6)	200 mg	500 mg
Folic Acid	1000 micrograms	none known
Vitamin B_{12}	3000 micrograms	none known
Calcium	1500 mg	more than 2500 mg
Magnesium	700 mg	none known
Chromium	1000 mcg	none known
Iron	65 mg	100 mg
Selenium	200 mcg	910 mcg
Zinc	30 mg	60 mg

*No adverse effects have been noted at this level.

SOURCE: John N. Hathcock, Vitamin and Mineral Safety, Council of Responsible Nutrition, Washington, D.C. (Hathcock, J.N., American Journal of Clinical Nutrition, 66:427–37, 1997) Copyright: Council for Responsible Nutrition. Reprinted with permission.

supplements at any age—they are extremely safe. But for sure, you should take B_{12} after age fifty (when atrophic gastritis could set in).

How much? Dr. Lindenbaum recommended that people past fifty take 500 to 1,000 micrograms of B_{12} a day. Dr. Robert Russell at Tufts University, also an expert on B_{12}, says all older people should take B_{12} supplements. He advises 1,000 micrograms daily, even 2000 micrograms if necessary to overcome severe malabsorption or advanced atrophic gastritis. B_{12} is considered remarkably safe even at high doses. In fact, there have never been any reports of adverse effects from B_{12} at any dose. However, some experts set 3000 micrograms daily as the top safe dose.

Thiamin:
A Psychiatric "Drug"

Not getting enough thiamin regularly can disrupt brain function. Your body keeps only small stores of thiamin around, so if you don't get it regularly in food or supplements, your brain can get in trouble after only a few weeks of deprivation. Severe deficiencies of thiamin lead to brain damage, including something called Korsakoff's psychosis (loss of memory, apathy, dementia) found most commonly among nutritionally-famished alcoholics.

> **BRAIN ALERT:** *A lack of thiamin is alarmingly widespread.*
> * *About 40 percent of older Americans brought to hospitals have a thiamin deficiency, according to a 1999 study. One reason: Many are taking diuretic drugs that interfere with metabolism of thiamin.*
> * *Some 22 percent of young men and 20 percent of young women showed borderline or fully deficient intakes of thiamin in a 1996 British study.*
> * *Recent autopsies in Australia found that 2.8 percent of the population had distinct signs of brain damage of the type caused by thiamin deficiency.*

MOOD CONTROL
It's well known that a lack of thiamin can ruin your mood, according to a string of studies dating back to the 1940s. In a recent study of older Irish women, fully 65 percent were either deficient or marginal in blood levels of thiamin. After a six-week regimen of taking 10 milligrams of thi-

amin a day, the women definitely were less fatigued and had greater feelings of well-being.

Too little thiamin also lowers the spirits of younger people. A recent German study of 1081 young men found 23 percent low in thiamin. They were more apt to be introverted, inactive, fatigued, with low self-confidence, and diminished mood. When they took 3 milligrams of thiamin a day for two months in a double-blind test, they became more sociable and happier.

"The first response to a thiamin-deficient diet is an inability to concentrate, confusion of thought, uncertainty of memory, anorexia, irritability, and depression." —R. D. Williams, *Archives of Internal Medicine*, 1942

THIAMIN AND DYSFUNCTIONAL BRAINS

The detrimental effects of marginal thiamin deficiencies on the brain has been known for decades. In the early 1940s, pioneering psychologist-researcher Ruth Harrell, then at Teachers College, Columbia University in New York, extensively investigated the impact of vitamins on children, especially those with poor diets. In one double-blind study, she gave thiamin supplements to eleven-year-old children in an orphanage who consumed a mere one milligram of thiamin daily. After a year, the children taking thiamin showed increases in reaction time, intelligence, visual acuity, memory, and reaction times.

More recently, in the 1980s, Derrick Lonsdale, M.D., then a researcher at the Cleveland Clinic Foundation specializing in pediatric and adolescent medicine, did red blood cell studies on more than 1000 patients, children and adults, and confirmed that 28 percent had a thiamin deficiency, often of long standing. The patients had been referred for various behavioral problems, such as hyper-activity, learning disability, tantrums, erratic temper, violent mood swings, depression, anxiety, and sleep problems.

Dr. Lonsdale routinely gave them a multivitamin-mineral supplement containing high doses of B vitamins, including thiamin, or thiamin alone. Their blood-cell thiamin became normal, usually within a few months, in nearly all cases. Remarkably, as their thiamin deficiency cleared up, their symptoms lessened or completely vanished. This, he said, "strongly suggests that the symptoms were caused by disturbed brain chemistry" of a type long attributed to thiamin deficiency. Lonsdale suggested that such patients actually had the early symptoms of beriberi, a nerve-damaging condition due to severe thiamin deficiency. He also concluded that "the surprisingly high incidence of abnormal tests revealed a widespread nutritional deficiency in the United States."

He also tied the thiamin deficiency and behavioral problems to a long-time diet of "junk food," including "empty" calorie soft drinks. In animals, he says, a high-sugar diet along with a thiamin deficiency is extremely threatening to brain functioning.

Undeniably, a lack of thiamin is common in youngsters. One British survey found that fully 49 percent of adolescent girls and 19 percent of boys consumed but one milligram of thiamin daily, suggesting a widespread deficiency severe enough to "cause psychological dysfunction," in the words of Dr. David Benton.

Dr. Benton recently showed that a supplement of nine vitamins raised mood in a group of 129 young healthy men and women. After a year they said they felt more "agreeable" than those taking a dummy pill. The women also said they felt more "composed" and that their mental health had improved. Not surprisingly, as their vitamin blood status rose, so did their moods and general mental health, indicating some deficiencies before the supplements.

Of all vitamins in the supplement, thiamin turned out to be the most formidable booster of mood, notably in women, Dr. Benton concluded. More surprising, he even found that an extra dose of thiamin may improve brain functioning and make you feel better—even if you are *not* technically deficient in thiamin. In a double-blind test of 120 women, average age twenty, all showed normal blood levels of thiamin. Nevertheless, Dr. Benton wondered whether an extra high dose of 50 milligrams of thiamin daily would have an impact on mood. It did. Thiamine takers said they were more clear-headed, composed, and energetic than before. They also had faster reaction times and made quicker decisions on a specific mental performance test. On the most difficult part of the test, the average microsecond reaction times of the thiamin takers quickened by about 13 percent, whereas reaction times of the placebo group remained about the same. The extra thiamin, however, did not improve memory in those with normal thiamin. Other research suggests it does improve memory in those who are thiamin deficient.

This does not mean everyone should take such super-high doses of thiamin. But it clearly indicates that the standard "normal" levels for thiamin may be insufficient for universal top brain functioning. The "normal" amounts that prevent overt symptoms of brain malfunction may not be enough to push the brain to its optimal feel-good and performance peaks.

BOTTOM LINE: *Taking thiamin improves brain functioning even in normal healthy women who have no overt signs of a deficiency.*

How could thiamin have such a powerful effect on the brain? According to Philip Langlais, Ph.D., professor of psychology at University of California, San Diego, Medical School, as quoted recently in *Psychology Today*, "A thiamin deficiency hampers the brain's ability to use glucose, decreasing energy available for mental activities. It also overexcites neurons so that they fire endlessly, poop out, and die.

"If you are even marginally deficient in thiamin," said Langlais, "you may be slowing down your brain power."

How much? Even the amount of thiamin in multivitamin supplements should be enough to prevent a deficiency. Some experts favor 25 milligrams a day to be sure. Even in high doses thiamin seems harmless, but experts put a "safe dose" at no more than 50 milligrams per day.

Niacin:
A Universal Memory Pill

Since niacin (also known as nicotinic acid, niacinamide, and nicotinamide) is such a common vitamin, found in virtually all supplements, few people realize its powers in the brain. For one thing, it is one of the primary boosters of energy production in the tiny factories of the cell, the mitochondria. This gives it a special place in brain protection, because if energy runs down, brain cells function less efficiently; also more free radical damage accumulates in the genes of the cell, potentially leading to its disability and death.

Small wonder that studies find niacin can have profound consequences for brain functioning.

Niacin may help improve memory in adults of any age. Dutch research psychologists at the Free University in Amsterdam tested megadoses of two forms of nicotinic acid on ninety-six healthy adults. Some took the real vitamin, some a placebo for eight weeks. Researchers tested their short-term, long-term, and sensory memories before and after they took the pills.

Conclusion: Niacin boosted memory performance by 10 to 40 percent over placebo. It worked in young brains, middle-aged brains, and elderly brains, boosting short-term, long-term, and sensory memory. Researchers theorize that niacin improves the transmission of electrical impulses between neurons, improving short-term memory circuits. In the elderly, it also facilitated long-term consolidation of memory, perhaps by encouraging synthesis of proteins needed to convert memory from short-term to long-term.

How does it work?

Nicotinamide is one of the nutrients known to stimulate energy generation in the cell's mitochondria. There's considerable evidence that the vitamin fights free radicals. It can prevent damage to and help repair free-radical-inflicted DNA injuries. Further, it can protect neurons of the substantia nigra, the part of the brain affected by Parkinson's disease, from damage induced by free-radical-generating neurotoxins.

In one dramatic experiment, Harvard researcher Flint Beal was able to diminish brain cell damage like that in Parkinson's and Alzheimer's diseases by using niacin. He found that adding niacin to the antioxidant coenzyme Q10 helped prevent mitochondrial brain cell destruction when coQ10 alone was ineffective.

NIACIN AND SCHIZOPHRENIA?

Although it's controversial, some doctors have used B vitamins, notably niacin, to treat schizophrenia. Its most vigorous advocate is Abram Hoffer, M.D., Ph.D., a practitioner of "orthomolecular" medicine and president of the Canadian Schizophrenia Organization, who has used niacin to treat schizophrenia for nearly fifty years in over 4,000 patients. Dr. Hoffer says the first patient who received niacin in 1952 improved within a month and became symptom-free in two years.

He insists that after two years of such orthomolecular treatment, "over 90 percent will be well, none will be worse, and none will have tardive dyskinesia" (a nerve damage from pharmaceutical drugs). His typical dose, which he says most patients must take for a lifetime: 1500 to 6000 milligrams of niacin (niacinamide or nicotinamide) daily in three divided doses. He also often adds 3000 mg vitamin C, 250 to 500 mg B_6, plus an assortment of other minerals if needed. He also advises patients to forgo processed sugary junk foods and any food to which they are allergic, and to eat essential fatty acids—omega–3 fatty acids, fish oil, and flaxseed oil.

> **BOTTOM LINE:** *Although the medical establishment finds little merit in niacin as a treatment for schizophrenia, it might be worth a try with proper medical supervision, say some experts, considering the difficulty of treating the disorder.*

How much? High doses of niacin in the form of nicotinic acid should only be taken under a doctor's supervision, because of the potential danger of adverse effects, including liver damage. Most adverse reactions to nicotinic acid, usually used to lower blood cholesterol, have happened from doses of 2000 to 6000 milligrams daily. Experts say the minimum dose for adverse effects from another form of niacin, nicotinamide, is 3000 milligrams per day.

A dose of 125 milligrams of niacin daily should be enough to protect normal brains.

Vitamin E:
Super Brain Pill

It's an alarming prospect, but true. Without sufficient vitamin E, the fatty parts of your brain are more apt to turn rancid, causing monumental disturbances in the normal functioning of neurons. The brain is mostly fat, making it extremely susceptible to fat-spoiling free radicals, and there is only one antioxidant, vitamin E, that dwells exclusively in the fatty part of cell membranes and thus can do constant battle with such free radicals on their home turf. That's the main reason many researchers believe vitamin E has the greatest proven record so far of all vitamins for protecting brain cells against breakdown due to normal "wear and tear" free radical attacks as well as degeneration caused by specific diseases, such as Alzheimer's. Evidence from autopsies show that deficiencies of vitamin E causes axons of nerve cells to degenerate and the cerebellum to shrink.

Vitamin E has many powers. But probably greatest is its strong antioxidant power to protect fat in cell membranes from undergoing "lipid peroxidation"—another word for rancidity—caused by free-radical chemicals. This "lipid peroxidation" also leads to clogged and hardened blood vessels everywhere, including those of the brain as well as the heart. Vitamin E is unique in that it can squelch ferocious free radical "chain reactions" that start with just one molecule and rage like wildfire through the body and brain, spreading rancidity and destroying cell after cell until stopped. "Vitamin E is like a cellular fire extinguisher," says one researcher, that snuffs out such biological rampages. Nowhere is this vitamin E protection more critical than in high-fat membranes of brain cells that must remain intact for the swift and accurate transmission of messages. Damaged or rancid membranes emit garbled messages, manifested as memory loss and other intellectual failures.

Indeed, the first sign of a vitamin E deficiency is a neurological problem.

EXCITING FACT: Vitamin E is the first nonprescription agent chosen for large scale human tests by the National Institute on Aging to determine if it slows memory loss in middle-aged persons, and prevents the onset of Alzheimer's disease. Results are expected in 2002.

BRAIN RESEARCHERS TAKE VITAMIN E

"I take 1000 IUs of vitamin E a day," says D. Allan Butterfield, a leading brain researcher and chemistry professor at the University of Kentucky's Sanders-Brown Center on Aging. He has studied vitamin E's ability to neutralize free radicals.

"I take 800 IUs of vitamin E daily," says Carl Cotman, director of the Institute of Brain Aging and Dementia at the University of California, Irvine.

"I take 400 IU of vitamin E daily," says Dr. Mark Mattson of the University of Kentucky's Sanders-Brown Center on Aging.

"I take 500 IU of natural vitamin E," says Dr. Lester Packer, Ph.D., world authority on antioxidants at the University of California at Berkeley.

FOUR WAYS VITAMIN E SAVES YOUR BRAIN

- Vitamin E neutralizes free radicals that damage the outer membranes of neurons, wrecking their ability to transmit messages, as well as the membranes of energy factories within cells, called mitochondria, that are key to a well-functioning brain.
- Vitamin E helps regulate message transmission *within* cells as well as between cells. This newly discovered so-called "second messenger system" is critical in directing and controlling activity of neurotransmitters once they enter the nerve cell.
- Vitamin E has immune-related benefits that reduce cell-damaging inflammation that is increasingly considered a primary villain in brain disease, including strokes and dementia.
- Vitamin E reduces clogging of blood vessels that are the conduits of life for brain cells by delivering oxygen. A primary cause of brain oxygen starvation and stroke is a blocked carotid (neck) artery. Plaque-filled small capillaries in the brain also cause oxygen starvation, ruptured cerebral vessels, and so-called mini-strokes. Vitamin E fights plaque buildup and promotes vascular flexibility.

THE MIND-BLOWING ALZHEIMER'S STUDY

Alzheimer's is agonizingly difficult to treat, and pharmaceutical drugs can have horrendous side effects. Yet, plain old vitamin E matched a prescription drug in treating Alzheimer's and was far safer. That's the conclusion of a study, bearing the names of six prestigious universities including Harvard, Columbia, and the University of California and published in one of the top mainstream medical journals in the world, *The New England Journal of Medicine,* in April 1997.

As a result, the American Psychiatric Association now recommends vitamin E, as well as certain prescription drugs such as Cognex and Aricept, as treatment for individuals diagnosed with mild or moderate dementia or Alzheimer's disease.

In the two-year study, 341 patients with moderately severe Alzheimer's randomly took either selegiline (a drug prescribed for Parkinson's and thought beneficial for Alzheimer's), or 1000 IU of synthetic vitamin E twice a day, or both vitamin E and the drug, or a placebo sugar pill.

The conclusion: Vitamin E delayed progression of Alzheimer's in more than half of those who took it, whereas most placebo takers continued to deteriorate. Vitamin E also slightly beat out selegiline and, oddly, was even better alone than when combined with the drug.

Specifically, vitamin E (and the drug) decreased functional breakdown in Alzheimer's patients—the ability to perform activities of daily living—by about 25 percent. Further, vitamin E takers survived longer and avoided institutionalization longer. Only 26 percent on vitamin E had to enter a nursing home during the study compared with 33 percent on the drug and 39 percent on placebo. Thus, vitamin E allowed patients to stay at home for an extra seven months before going to a nursing home. "No other treatments have shown a similar ability to delay important milestones in Alzheimer's disease," proclaimed the National Institute on Aging.

Researchers speculate vitamin E worked by increasing functioning and/or survival of certain brain cells, possibly by protecting them from destructive rancidity or oxidation. Interestingly, the study used synthetic instead of natural vitamin E. The results would probably have been even more impressive with natural vitamin E, says antioxidant expert Dr. Lester Packer.

> **BOTTOM LINE:** *Taking 2000 IU of alpha-tocopherol vitamin E daily delayed key signs of the progression of Alzheimer's disease, including the ability to bathe and dress, the need for institutionalization, and survival time.*

The big question for most Americans: Will taking vitamin E help prevent or slow down brain degeneration and the onset of Alzheimer's? Theoretically, it should, say many brain researchers who themselves are taking vitamin E to protect their own brains from deterioration. The National Institute on Aging thinks it's a good possibility, too. They are testing the theory on a group of 720 Americans, ages fifty-five to ninety, who have been diagnosed with "mild cognitive impairment," called MCI, meaning they score at the low end of normal for their age on memory tests. According to Dr. Leon Thal, principal investigator for the new study and chairman of neurosciences at the University of California, San Diego, about 75 percent of people with such cognitive impairment are expected to develop Alzheimer's. "Alzheimer's is not a sudden event, like falling down," he says. It comes on gradually and mild cognitive impairment, called MCI, is an early warning sign. In one study, 12 per cent of patients with MCI developed Alzheimer's within a year, compared with only 1 or 2 percent of healthy individuals.

Investigators hope vitamin E will delay the progression from MCI to full-blown Alzheimer's better than a placebo or the drug Aricept. The study will use a 1000 IU daily dose of synthetic alpha tocopherol for the first six weeks, and 2,000 IU daily after that.

In the meantime, there's plenty of reason to make you want to take vitamin E to protect your brain, especially if you are approaching middle age.

VITAMIN E TAKERS DIDN'T GET ALZHEIMER'S

A striking new double-blind study did show your risk of Alzheimer's goes way down if you take vitamin E. A team of researchers from Chicago's Rush Institute for Healthy Aging and Harvard Medical School studied 633 individuals age sixty-five or older, giving them memory tests and carefully examining what vitamins they took, especially vitamins E and C.

More than four years later, investigators reevaluated the mental functioning of the group through neurological examinations and testing. Ninety-one were diagnosed with "probable Alzheimer's." However, the stunning finding was that not a single person among the twenty-seven who took vitamin E supplements developed Alzheimer's; expected cases were four, or about 15 percent. Moreover, no one among the twenty-three who took vitamin C supplements developed Alzheimer's, either, although again 15 percent would be expected.

How much did they take? From 200 to 800 IU of vitamin E daily. Typical doses were 400 IU of vitamin E or 500 milligrams of vitamin C daily, standard amounts in separate supplements. It's important to note that taking multivitamin supplements containing low doses of vitamin E (usually 30 IU) and vitamin C (60 milligrams) did *not* reduce the odds of Alzheimer's. Such multivitamin users in the study were just as likely to develop Alzheimer's as those who took no vitamins! There is probably too little E and C in conventional multivitamin pills to protect the brain, researchers said.

Imagine! The number of individuals taking vitamin E or vitamin C who developed Alzheimer's was zero—"the strongest result possible," as researchers noted. To put it another compelling way: Whether you take vitamin E or C could actually predict whether Alzheimer's is in your future!

> **BRAIN ALERT:** *About thirty percent of Americans have a known deficiency of vitamin E, according to government statistics.*

DRAMATIC BRAIN IMAGES OF VITAMIN E PROTECTION

What if you could get a secret look at your own brain tissue to see how it is holding up under everyday damage from years of free-radical attacks and other biological assaults? What if you had compelling visual evidence suggesting that vitamin E could help protect your brain from subtle cumulative damage? Austrian researchers Reinhold Schmidt, M.D., and colleagues at the Karl-Franzens University of Graz, have produced such remarkable new brain scan images, showing that subtle brain damage is directly tied to low amounts of vitamin E in the blood. The investigators used magnetic resonance imaging (MRI) to spot signs of subtle brain damage in 355 normal volunteers ages forty-five to seventy-five. In a word, they took dramatic pictures of brains on their way to ruin.

The type of brain pathology the researchers focused on is known as "white matter hyperintensities"—tiny abnormalities or injuries in brain tissue, suggesting small vessel disease in cerebral white matter. It's common in the elderly, evident in 40 to 50 percent of elderly brains. Although it is "benign" in that it produces no noticeable symptoms in normal older people, it nevertheless is a sign of blood vessel damage and cognitive impairment and a predictor of worse things to come. One possible cause: vascular disease, including high blood pressure. Another logical cause: perpetual brain cell battering and oxidation by free-radical chemicals over many years.

If hordes of free radicals are a cause, one would expect that the more extensive the white matter injuries, the weaker the body's antioxidant forces at combating the free radicals. To test that theory, the Austrian researchers measured ten naturally occurring antioxidants in the subjects' bloodstreams. The results were stunning.

Low levels of blood lycopene (from tomatoes) were indicative of increased brain damage. But most striking was a link with vitamin E. Those with the least blood vitamin E had *seven times or 700 percent* more early brain matter damage than those with the highest blood levels of vitamin E. Although the exact mechanisms of the damage are uncertain, vitamin E appears to keep it in check, protecting the aging brain. When a stark visual picture shows that your brain looks less bruised and beaten up just because you have more vitamin E in your veins, it's enough to make anybody reach for the vitamin E.

In another study of 1769 healthy subjects ages fifty to seventy-five years, Dr. Schmidt's group found that those with the lowest vitamin E blood levels scored worst on a rating scale that measures dementia, another word for failure of intellectual functions. Yet, they did not exhibit overt symptoms of mental decline. The connection held true regardless of sex, education, smoking, or blood cholesterol levels.

Stop the Surgery, Give Me Vitamin E

One of the biggest causes of stroke is a blockage in the carotid artery of the neck leading to the brain. Plaque builds up, the artery narrows, and the supply of blood and oxygen to brain cells is cut off. Often doctors can spot the impending carotid disaster through ultrasound pictures of the neck. The challenge then: how to remove the gunk, opening the artery. One way is by surgery, a procedure called carotid endarterectomy, which carries some risk to the patient.

But surprising new research has recently discovered another utterly safe method: A specific form of vitamin E can help clean out blocked carotid arteries! It seems incredible, but it has been documented in a remarkable ongoing five-year double-blind study by cardiologist Marvin Bierenbaum and colleagues of the Kenneth L. Jordan Heart Research Foundation in Montclair, New Jersey. For four years, researchers gave fifty patients, ages forty-nine to eighty-three, with severe carotid narrowing (stenosis) either a vitamin E combination of about 100 milligrams of alpha tocopherol plus 240 milligrams of tocotrienols (another form of vitamin E), or a placebo. The degree of narrowing of the carotid arteries ranged from 15 to 79 percent. Many had already had a nondisabling stroke or a transient ischemic attack (TIA), a warning sign of stroke. Most continued their regular medications, including aspirin.

Ultrasound scans recorded the state of the carotid arteries at six months, twelve months, and then annually. Within six months, the benefits of vitamin E were evident. After four years, the consequences of *not* taking vitamin E were frightening. The amazing results: Carotid artery clogging regressed, or diminished in *40 percent* of those on the vitamin E mixture. Blood flow through the carotid arteries also improved. Only 12 percent got worse; the others had no change. In contrast, fully 60 percent on the placebo (five times as many as on the vitamin E) suffered progressive narrowing and clogging of the carotid arteries; in some it was quite marked. Interestingly, in the first part of the study, vitamin E derived from palm oil opened up carotid arteries without lowering cholesterol. It apparently worked its miracle of sweeping away plaque primarily by boosting antioxidant activity and modifying blood coagulation factors, say researchers. A later phase of the study did find that tocotrienol-rich bran oil lowered bad LDL cholesterol by 21 percent.

In any event, the study clearly demonstrates that vitamin E, mostly as tocotrienols, somehow scrubbed down the artery walls, washing away plaque, claims Dr. Bierenbaum. He calls it "a breakthrough study," proving there is an "alternative to surgery." He also notes that taking vitamin E could prevent your carotid arteries from becoming blocked in the first place.

It's important to note that Dr. Bierenbaum uses some ordinary vitamin E (alpha tocopherol), but primarily other types of vitamin E called tocotrienols, extracted from palm oil or rice bran oil. He credits the tocotrienols for most of the regression in the carotid arteries.

Vitamin E as Stroke Antidote

Considering vitamin E's ability to partly restore carotid arteries to health, perhaps it's not surprising to find evidence that the vitamin deters strokes. A new study showed that a large group of older people (average age sixty-nine) who took in the most vitamin E, primarily from supplements, slashed their risk of having an ischemic (blood-clot) stroke, the most common type, by an astonishing 53 percent. Surprisingly, the protective dose of vitamin E was very small—from 42 to 72 international units (IU) a day. That compared with stroke victims who averaged only 27 units of E daily. Most multivitamins contain around 30 units of E, although most experts recommend taking 400 IUs a day. The tiny amount of vitamin E in food was not enough to ward off strokes, researchers concluded. The study, part of the Northern Manhattan Stroke Study, was headed by Dr. Ralph L. Sacco at Columbia University.

VITAMIN E WARDS OFF PARKINSON'S DISEASE
Since free-radical damage to the brain is considered a culprit in Parkinson's disease, it makes sense that eating lots of antioxidants might help prevent the disorder. Dutch researchers at Erasmus University Medical School in Rotterdam have found evidence supporting the theory. They surveyed 5324 individuals, ages fifty-five to ninety-five. Those ingesting the most vitamin E were least likely to develop Parkinson's. High vitamin C and beta carotene in food also showed some protection, but not nearly as much as vitamin E.

However, giving high doses of vitamin E to treat Parkinson's has been only mildly effective. What this means, say experts, is that vitamin E and perhaps other antioxidants may work to help prevent brain disorders and may even help forestall progress in the early stages, but are less effective once the disease is advanced. "Prevention is more powerful than treatment," says vitamin E expert Andreas Papas, Ph.D., at Eastman Kodak (a supplier of raw materials for vitamin supplements) and author of a recent book, *The Vitamin E Factor*.

WHAT TYPE VITAMIN E?
Vitamin E comes in eight different chemical forms—four tocopherols and four tocotrienols (designated as alpha, beta, gamma, and delta), as found naturally in food. The

most common, put into most vitamin preparations, is alpha tocopherol, either synthetic or natural. Of this form, many experts favor "natural" vitamin E, noted on labels as d-alpha tocopherol. However, other types of vitamin E, particularly gamma tocopherol and gamma tocotrienol, also promise brain protection. Gamma, too, is a potent antioxidant protector of cell membranes, and may have special powers against degenerative brain diseases. One reason: Gamma vitamin E is uniquely potent in neutralizing a class of free radicals known as "nitrogen" free radicals that are particularly lethal to nerve cells. These nitrogen radicals are primary culprits in brain diseases, including Alzheimer's. Thus, many leading antioxidant researchers now say you need a full range of vitamin E, including both alpha and gamma types of vitamin E, as well as tocotrienols to fully protect the brain.

When choosing vitamin E for brain protection, Dr. Packer advises looking for "mixed" tocopherols that include gamma as well as alpha. You can also buy tocotrienols alone or in mixtures with tocopherols—for example, one new vitamin E supplement contains 400 IU of tocopherols and 400 milligrams of tocotrienols.

How much? Four to five hundred IUs of natural vitamin E daily is usually considered adequate for good antioxidant protection. Take no more than 1000 IU of vitamin E daily, except on a doctor's advice. The potential hazard: excessively thin blood, notably if you also take anticoagulants. Vitamin E has been reported to accentuate bleeding in a dose of 800 IU daily when taken with a blood thinner, such as Coumadin.

BRAIN MESSAGES FROM THE LABORATORY

For decades, scientists have known from studies of laboratory animals that a vitamin E deficiency strikes the nervous system with a vengeance. Vitamin E-deficient rats and their offspring often suffer paralysis and "nutritional muscular dystrophy." Rhesus monkeys, as well as chicks and rats, fed vitamin E-deficient diets develop ataxia (loss of balance), weakness, and other neurologic disturbances. Giving animals high vitamin E doses has reduced the damage to hippocampus cells following a stroke; and pretreating animals with vitamin E speeds recovery of motor function after spinal cord injury.

Simply giving animals twice the amount of vitamin E in their diets over a period of time substantially reduced the amount of brain damage following a brain hemorrhage or stroke. Thus, some experts suspect that modest doses of vitamin E supplements—100 to 400 IU daily—may help protect humans from neurological damage after a stroke.

Vitamin C:
Brain Saver

It's smart to take vitamin C, and it may make you even smarter. Vitamin C is a very strong antioxidant that researchers have only recently discovered passes readily through the blood-brain barrier; is concentrated in high levels in brain tissue; contributes to the creation of neuro-transmitters, such as dopamine; and protects cells from free-radical damage.

That's why numerous studies show that higher amounts of vitamin C in the bloodstream boost cognitive performance apparently at all ages and protect against age-related brain degeneration, including Alzheimer's disease and strokes.

ACTIVATES YOUNG BRAINS
Although many vitamins may help boost brain power, vitamin C often stands out. For example, British investigators found that adolescent boys ages thirteen to fourteen with the highest blood levels of vitamin C had the highest scores on nonverbal IQ tests. Vitamin C is also known to boost blood levels of glutathione, another antioxidant linked to higher scores on IQ tests.

VITAMIN C ORANGE JUICE DRIVES UP IQ SCORES
In an early fascinating study, two psychologists from Texas Woman's University in Denton, Texas, in 1960 showed that drinking orange juice could boost IQ scores in school-children. Researchers argued that one reason kids from

lower socioeconomic levels score lower on IQ tests may be an undetected nutritional deficiency that hinders mental growth and performance and that the condition may not be permanent, but reversible.

So they devised a test. They gave 236 schoolchildren from kindergarten to ninth grade and 115 university students age-appropriate IQ tests. They also analyzed vitamin C blood levels and classified children as high or low. As theorized, they discovered that kids with the highest blood vitamin C generally had higher IQ scores by five to ten points. Next question: Could they raise IQ scores in low-C kids by giving them vitamin-C rich orange juice at school for six months? Yes; it worked. When retested after six months of drinking orange juice at school (the amount was not specified), kids with originally high-vitamin C blood showed very little improvement in IQ scores. However, average IQ scores in low-vitamin C kids shot up about four points! Further, IQ scores generally rose along with blood vitamin C concentrations.

Researchers suggested that the extra orange juice and/or vitamin C boosted brain "alertness" or "sharpness" in those who needed it, supporting the idea that high vitamin C kids already functioned at near maximum brain capacity, while the lower C group functioned below maximum brain capacity.

VITAMIN C VS. MENTAL DECLINE

Vitamin C is especially essential for preserving aging brains. You can predict the vitality of your mental function as you age by how much vitamin C you take in, according to recent research. The more vitamin C, the less apt you are to lose your mind. Particularly impressive evidence comes from Australian researchers at the University of Sydney. In a study of 117 older persons they found that those who took vitamin C supplements were only 40 percent as apt to have severe cognitive impairment as non-vitamin C takers, as judged by scores on the highly valid Mini-Mental State Examination. This was true regardless of educational level. When supplement users also ate a high vitamin C diet, the odds of intellectual decline dropped even more—to only 32 percent.

A recent Swiss study of older people (ages sixty-five to ninety-four) showed that those with the highest blood levels of vitamin C performed best on tests of various forms of memory.

VITAMIN C AS STROKE FIGHTER

A primary way vitamin C seems to deter mental decline is by combating cerebrovascular disease, namely strokes. British researchers at the University of Southampton recently studied 921 men and women age sixty-five and over. They found that those with the most vitamin C in their diets and in their blood had the best cognitive function and the lowest risk of fatal strokes. Subjects who took in more than 45 milligrams of vitamin C daily showed only half as much cognitive impairment as those who took in less than 28 milligrams of vitamin C daily. Further, those who scored lowest on tests of intellectual functioning were nearly three times as likely to die of a stroke as those who had no evidence of cognitive impairment. The evidence points decidedly to vitamin C as the link between cognitive function and strokes. Those were with the least dietary and blood vitamin C were also three times more apt to die of a stroke than those with the most. In fact, *low vitamin C* was as big a risk factor for deadly stroke as high diastolic blood pressure.

The inevitable conclusions: "A subclinical deficiency" of vitamin C predicts impaired cognitive function in older people. A high vitamin C intake protects against both cognitive impairment and cerebrovascular disease. A large proportion of cognitive decline in the elderly is vascular in origin."

Similarly, a large-scale Swiss study of nearly 3000 middle-aged men showed that those with low blood vitamin C and beta-carotene had four times the risk of a fatal stroke.

How does vitamin C fight strokes? One way: It suppresses abnormalities, including clogging, in the carotid artery that signal mental decline and strokes. Researcher Stephen Kritchevsky at the University of Tennessee recently found that women over age fifty-five who took vitamin C supplements had carotid arteries with less thickening of the walls—that is, larger openings for blood and oxygen to flow through on the way to the brain. This is important, because new research identifies thickened carotid artery walls as a leading predictor of memory and cognitive decline after age sixty-five.

Vitamin C also regulates vascular function—the dilation and contraction of arteries and blood flow—in ways that discourage traveling blood clots that can block cerebral vessels. Vitamin C for one thing makes plaque more "stable" so bits are less apt to break off and form clots.

STROKE DYNAMICS AND VITAMIN C

Further, if you have a stroke, you may suffer less damage if your blood contains high amounts of vitamin C. That's a clue scientists have picked up from hibernating animals. During a stroke, the cutoff of oxygen and glucose causes massive brain cell destruction. Moreover, as blood flow resumes in a rush, there is a second wave of destruction of cells trying to recover from the attack. It is called "reperfusion injury," and can be as frightful as the initial assault on the brain. The cause is the sudden reinfusion of blood, oxygen, and mainly free-radical chemicals to the brain.

Scientists have discovered this also happens in hibernating animals when they wake up after a long sleep. But why don't they suffer severe brain damage when they are aroused from their torpor? Margaret E. Rice of New York University Medical Center may have a partial answer. During hibernation, squirrels' blood flow to the brain is reduced to a trickle, by 90 percent or more, she says. However, at the same time blood vitamin C soars 400 percent and vitamin C in the cerebrospinal fluid of the central nervous system doubles and remains high during the long sleep. Dr. Rice believes this vitamin C buildup is nature's way of protecting animals' brains from the surge of free radicals that comes when blood flow returns to normal and brain cells vigorously start burning oxygen again. In short, the vitamin C acts as a strong antioxidant to neutralize the free radical onslaught that would otherwise destroy brain tissue.

It's logical that high blood levels of vitamin C in humans whose brains are under attack from free radicals during a stroke might also reduce damage to brain cells, lessening the severity of a stroke.

How does vitamin C affect the brain? At least 400 medical articles have been published in answer to that question. Vitamin C's most obvious power is as an antioxidant. Leading researcher Lester Packer says vitamin C is one of the five most powerful "network" antioxidants, along with vitamin E, coenzyme Q10, lipoic acid, and glutathione. As an antioxidant, it protects brain cells from extensive damage by free radical assaults. For example, studies have shown that people with Alzheimer's disease have much lower levels of vitamin C in the cerebrospinal fluid than young healthy people. In one recent study not a single person developed Alzheimer's who had taken vitamin C supplements.

It's evident the brain considers vitamin C essential for optimal functioning, say experts, because it insists on keeping extremely high levels in brain cells. Animal studies show that vitamin C quickly and easily enters the brain. After injecting lab animals with vitamin C, scientists can detect vitamin C in their brains within minutes!

Vitamin C, however, is more than an antioxidant. It facilitates the transmission of messages through the brain. It can directly influence electrical impulses, the synthesis (the brain needs vitamin C to make dopamine and adrenaline) and release of neurotransmitters and their journey through cell synapses. In short, vitamin C is a prime player in the all-important connector sites of the brain that determine the quality and quantity of transmissions.

How much? A moderate dose of 500 to 1000 milligrams of vitamin C daily is thought to be sufficient to protect the brain. Some experts think even 200 milligrams may be enough.

Safety: Vitamin C is incredibly safe at very high doses. No toxicity has been detected at doses of 20,000 milligrams a day, the amount Dr. Linus Pauling took. You may experience loose bowel movements after taking high doses of vitamin C, but they subside when you lower the dose.

Brain Boosting Mineral: Selenium

The trace mineral selenium has a huge impact on brain function. Nerve cells must have selenium to produce glutathione, one of the brain's most important antioxidants. The brains of animals, for example, fed a low selenium diet make less glutathione. Such selenium-deprived brains also show disturbances in the activity of prominent neurotransmitters serotonin, dopamine, and adrenaline, signifying potential brain damage and dysfunction, according to recent research. Further blood levels of selenium drop as you age—by 7 percent after age sixty and 24 percent after age seventy-five, according to one study.

Low Selenium, Low Moods

Skimping on selenium does disturb human moods, possibly because of disruptions in neurotransmitter activity. U.S. Department of Agriculture researchers fed a group of young men either a low-selenium or high-selenium diet for about three-and-a-half months. The high selenium diet raised men's spirits considerably. They said they felt more clear-headed, elated, agreeable, composed, confident, and energetic. Further, the more selenium in the men's red blood cells, the better they felt. USDA research psychologist James G. Penland, who conducted the study, said the extra selenium lifted the men's moods even though they had no signs of selenium deficiency. This implies that Americans do not eat enough selenium for optimal well-being, but are unaware of a problem. In other words, undetected subclinical deficiencies may be ruining our moods. The study's high-selenium diet contained 220 micrograms daily, the low-selenium diet 33 micrograms. A typical American diet contains from 40 to 60 micrograms of selenium per day.

Foods high in selenium: grains, garlic, meat, seafood—especially tuna, swordfish and oysters—and Brazil nuts. Eating a Brazil nut is like taking a selenium pill, say experts. A shelled Brazil nut averages 12 to 25 micrograms a nut. If you buy them in the shell and extract them, the nut contains about 100 micrograms of selenium.

TAKE SELENIUM, FEEL BETTER

British psychologist David Benton also found "marked improvement in mood" in fifty subjects, ages fourteen to seventy-four, who took a 100 microgram selenium pill daily for five weeks—even though they had no obvious signs of

---

DOES SELENIUM EXPLAIN GARLIC AS MOOD FOOD?

Several researchers have reported that garlic elevates mood. Garlic's high selenium content may be one explanation. Indian researchers testing garlic's benefits for heart attack patients have noted a favorable side effect: better mood and more energy. French scientist Dr. Gilles Fillion of the Pasteur Institute found that garlic promotes the release of feel-good serotonin. "I suspect garlic is antistress, antianxiety, and acts as a sort of antidepressant like Prozac, although with a much milder effect," he said. "Eating garlic may just make you feel better." In mice, Japanese researchers pronounced garlic extract 60 percent as effective as Valium in relieving stress.

deficiency. Some got a placebo, the others the real thing. Selenium takers, on a standard mood inventory test, felt strikingly more clear-headed, composed, energetic, elated, confident, agreeable—or conversely, less confused, anxious, tired, depressed, unsure, and hostile. Selenium's greatest benefit was reducing anxiety.

Researchers also noted that subjects who usually ate the least selenium benefited most from the supplement. Their mood scores shot up more than 40 percent after five weeks on the selenium supplement. Even those on relatively high selenium diets had a striking improvement—their mood scores jumped 25 percent. The explanation: A subclinical unsuspected selenium deficiency, manifested as low mood, was alleviated by the supplements.

It's not the first time selenium supplements have improved mental function. In one Dutch study, geriatric patients given selenium and vitamin E tablets had less anxiety, depression, and more mental alertness. Other research found that a mixture of selenium, zinc, and evening prim-rose oil improved mood and some aspects of mental function in a group of older people with memory loss.

How much? Experts advise taking 200 micrograms of selenium a day to protect your brain as well as discourage heart disease and cancer. But beware of high doses. Selenium is one of the few supplements that can be extremely toxic. Although toxicity may not kick in until you eat 2500 micrograms a day, there is no reason to exceed 200 micrograms of selenium daily in a supplement.

BOTTOM LINE: *Subtle, widespread deficiencies of selenium upset brain function, particularly lowering mood and raising anxiety. You must have adequate selenium for optimal brain functioning. The solution: a 200 microgram daily supplement.*

Lipoic Acid:
Number One
Super Antioxidant

One of the most formidable protectors of your brain is an antioxidant you may never have heard of. Dr. Lester Packer, professor of molecular and cell biology at the University of California at Berkeley, and one of the world's leading researchers on antioxidants, calls alpha-lipoic acid the "superantioxidant," closest to his vision of an "ideal" antioxidant if he were to design one. Indeed, in Dr. Packer's hierarchy of five so-called "network antioxidants"—designated as the mightiest among hundreds of antioxidants—he puts lipoic acid number one. Lipoic acid is "the most versatile and powerful" of all antioxidants, he declares. It is an incomparable brain antioxidant—the antioxidant's antioxidant.

Several things make it unique and universal, finds Dr. Packer. Because it is a small molecule it is one of the few substances that can readily penetrate the blood-brain barrier and be quickly taken up by brain tissue; thus, it goes directly to the aid and rescue of target cells under attack in the brain. "It is the only antioxidant that can easily get into the brain," he says.

Moreover, unlike any other antioxidant, it is both fat and water soluble because of its unique chemical structure, and thus able to work its miracles in both the watery and fatty portions of the cell, wherever it is most needed. No other antioxidant can do that. And there's more. Lipoic acid is the only antioxidant that can recycle or regenerate itself as well as all four other crucial antioxidants—vitamins E and C, glutathione, and coenzyme Q10. This means that when an antioxidant like vitamin E or C is exhausted and depleted, lipoic acid rushes in to restore it to its full antioxidant powers. It is also the only antioxidant that can reinvent itself as an antioxidant after it has expended itself fighting off free radical assaults.

Further, lipoic acid neutralizes the very type of free radical most apt to injure brain cells—nitrogen radicals, including nitric oxide. Most attention has been focused on defusing so-called ordinary oxygen radicals, but there is another type free radical that scientists have lately begun to focus on more intensely. It is the nitrogen free radical and it is particularly hazardous to brain cells.

Also critical, lipoic acid increases the efficiency of the energy factories of the cells—the mitochondria. With age, energy production in mitochondria declines, meaning they utilize oxygen and glucose less efficiently and produce more free radical damage. Dr. Bruce Ames and colleagues at the University of California, Berkeley, found that lipoic acid recharged energy levels in aged rats—in fact, it reversed the reduction of cellular energy in old rats by 50 percent! The rats' physical activity also picked up, returning them almost to the activity levels of young rats.

One other major talent of lipoic acid is that it helps control blood sugar and insulin levels and helps block formation of sugar-damaged proteins called AGEs (advanced glycation end products) that accelerate aging and occur in high levels in diabetics.

Lipoic acid is technically not a vitamin because your body can produce it, but production declines as you age and by middle age is not enough for full protection.

MEMORY CURE

Worried about declining memory? Lipoic acid may restore youthful memory. In dramatic experiments, German researchers at the Clinical Institute for Mental Health in Mannheim put lipoic acid in the drinking water of aged but otherwise healthy mice. Just like humans, animals tend to show signs of age-associated memory impairment as they grow older. And for the same probable reason: a lifetime of free-radical attacks on brain tissue. After two weeks, mice that drank both lipoic-acid-fortified water and plain drinking water were tested to see how well they could negotiate a maze; success depended on how well they remembered.

Sure enough, mice that got lipoic acid-spiked water did far better and displayed far better memories. In fact, some performed as well as or better than mice half their age, suggesting that lipoic acid's antioxidant activity drastically slowed brain deterioration, perhaps by preventing neuron losses and/or repairing faulty transmission systems.

What's also remarkable is how quickly lipoic acid worked its memory-restoring miracle—in only two weeks. In human terms that would be about a year-and-a-half for a seventy-five-year-old. Is it possible lipoic acid could work on human brains in such a short time—a mere year-and-a-half? "It might be possible, but it's quite unproven," says Dr. Packer. He also stresses that lipoic acid does not spur growth of new brain cells. It's believed lipoic acid boosts memory by rejuvenating the functioning of specific receptors on nerve cell membranes that control message transmissions throughout the brain.

Interestingly, lipoic acid did not improve memory in *young* animals. This suggests lipoic acid repairs and revitalizes worn-out circuits in aged brain cells, but does not create supra-normal performance in young, healthy neurons.

"Lipoic acid is the most powerful antioxidant known to man." —Lester Packer, professor of molecular and cell biology, University of California at Berkeley

PREVENTING STROKE DAMAGE

Lipoic acid may keep you from having a stroke—but if you have one, it may help limit the damage and speed your recovery, according to impressive animal evidence. Laboratory animals given lipoic acid recover quickly from strokes, says Dr. Packer. He induced strokes in rats by blocking the carotid artery that carries blood and oxygen to the brain. In such strokes, blood flow is disrupted, but then suddenly resumes as the blockage dissipates. That's the dangerous part of a stroke—during so-called reperfusion, when the oxygen rushes back into the brain. That rush provokes a burst of free radical formation in the brain of such magnitude that the brain's ordinary antioxidant defenses cannot handle it and are wiped out. As a result defenseless brain cells are injured and killed (during reperfusion), resulting in temporary or permanent damage and possibly death. This is the nature of stroke damage. In Dr. Packer's study, 80 percent of the rats died within a day after restoration of oxygen to the brain.

But what happens to such rats if you give them a shot of lipoic acid just before the blood and oxygen begin to flow normally back into the brain? "It's amazing, incredible," says Dr. Packer. In such an experiment, only 25 percent of the stroke animals given lipoic acid died and all the survivors fully recovered without a trace of damage. "There's no other antioxidant or drug that could perform such a feat of preventing stroke-related brain injury," says Dr. Packer.

Further, Dr. Packer's research proved that lipoic acid performed the magic by preventing free radical damage to vulnerable parts of the brain. An examination of the rats' brains revealed that those denied lipoic acid had extensive free-radical induced brain damage. Those given lipoic acid had normal brains devoid of the free radical damage usually seen after a stroke. Other researchers have found nearly identical rates of increased stroke survival due to treatment with lipoic acid.

So what can you make of this? Dr. Packer and other researchers suggest that lipoic acid might be used by physicians to treat stroke victims, lessening the reperfusion injury to the brain. There's also the likelihood that keeping your brain cells supplied with high amounts of lipoic acid might protect them from damage in case of stroke, because their antioxidant defenses are much stronger.

PROTECTS NERVE CELLS OF DIABETICS

High blood sugar and insulin levels are not kind to nerve cells. In fact, these two villains can attack and destroy nerve cells in diabetics. Such disturbance of the peripheral nervous system, known as diabetic neuropathy, is a major and painful complication for many with diabetes. Yet, lipoic acid has been used successfully for twenty-five years in Europe to treat diabetic neuropathy. High doses of lipoic acid—200 to 600 milligrams daily—have relieved symptoms markedly within two or three weeks, German investigators report. Indeed, lipoic acid can even stimulate regeneration of nerve fibers in those with diabetic neuropathy.

Further, lipoic acid improves insulin function or "sensitivity" and lowers blood sugar in Type 2 (adult-onset) diabetics, according to several studies by German researchers. The dose: 600 milligrams twice a day for four weeks. Prominent physicians in this country are now planning tests of lipoic acid to treat diabetes. It also seems likely, says Dr.

Packer, that taking lipoic acid prevents the onset of Type 2 diabetes by helping stabilize blood sugar and insulin levels.

THE GLUTATHIONE MIRACLE

There's another crucial way lipoic acid indirectly protects your brain. Lipoic acid is strongly connected to another important antioxidant called glutathione. This antioxidant is synthesized by the body, but it is extremely difficult to raise levels of glutathione in brain cells or even in blood cells. Taking glutathione orally won't do it, because most of it is destroyed by enzymes in the digestive tract before it can be absorbed and delivered to cells. Even if you inject glutathione into the bloodstream, it does not reach the brain.

However, there is one sure way to raise blood and brain levels of glutathione: Take lipoic acid. Lipoic acid in the bloodstream causes glutathione to soar in the brain, studies show. The lipoic acid molecule is small enough to slip through the blood-brain barrier, and once inside the brain, it mysteriously regenerates glutathione, something no other antioxidant can do.

In experiments, Dr. Packer found that adding lipoic acid to various types of animal and human cells in test tubes boosted production of glutathione by an astonishing 30 to 70 percent! Feeding lipoic acid to laboratory animals also quickly and significantly raised levels of glutathione in their organs and blood.

It's impossible to estimate how critical glutathione is in protecting cells from free radicals. Some have called it the "master antioxidant." Mainly it detoxifies the body. Studies show people with high levels of glutathione stay younger longer in all ways. Low levels of glutathione predict chronic diseases, including degenerative brain disorders and early death.

BOTTOM LINE: *The best way to make sure you have ultra-protective glutathione in brain cells is to take lipoic acid.*

DON'T DEPEND ON FOOD

You get little alpha lipoic acid in food. Of sixteen foods analyzed by Dr. Packer, spinach was the richest source by far. Next in line: beef kidney and heart, broccoli, beef liver, tomatoes, garden peas, Brussels sprouts, and rice bran. Bananas, orange peel, soybeans, and horseradish had none. Still, Dr. Packer says, you would have to eat more than fifteen pounds of spinach to get a mere two milligrams of lipoic acid, a tiny amount.

HOW MUCH TO TAKE?

Many experts favor a dose of 10 to 50 milligrams of lipoic acid a day for healthy people. Dr. Packer takes 100 milligrams daily, half in the morning and half in the late afternoon or evening. If you are diabetic, you may need more—200 to 600 milligrams daily. Consult your doctor. Lipoic acid is available over the counter in health food stores. The major distributor is the well-regarded Henkel Corporation, which is funding many double-blind studies on lipoic acid in this country. Lipoic acid is sold under several different brands.

Toxicity? None reported, even in high doses. However, doses over 100 milligrams could conceivably lower blood sugar too much in normal nondiabetic individuals.

Coenzyme Q10:
Mighty Brain Energizer

Coenzyme Q10 is essential as a brain booster and rejuvenator, helping protect your brain against "normal" aging and the serious brain diseases that accompany it.

If your brain cells run low on coenzyme Q10, also known as coQ10, energy production in the tiny furnaces of the neuron, the mitochondria, slows down, creating an energy crisis and dysfunction. Add to that increased onslaughts by hordes of free radicals intent on turning the fat in your nerve cell membranes rancid so message transmission is screwed up and the cell's survival is in peril. The stage is set for eventual catastrophe, even though it may be many years in the making: an erosion of brain integrity, intellectual decline, memory loss, motor disturbances, and the cluster of degenerative brain diseases, including Alzheimer's, Parkinson's, and ALS.

RUNNING ON EMPTY
Imagine trying to start your car, but the engine doesn't turn over and you discover the spark plugs are faulty. Without the spark, the engine is inoperative. The same thing happens in your brain if you lack coenzyme Q10. This remarkable antioxidant is "the cellular spark plug," says Dr. Lester Packer, that incites the tiny energy centers, the mitochondria, in nerve cells (and other cells), to churn out the vital chemical ATP (adenosine triphosphate) that fuels all life. Without coenzyme Q10, there is no spark to rev up the cell's energy production. It's not hard to imagine how sluggish

brain cells become without coQ10. Their energy engines are apt to misfire or fail totally. In a word, "you are running on empty," says Dr. Packer, or at the very least on low-octane fuel.

Essentially, coQ10 molecules are the workers within the micro-energy factories, or mitochondria, that shuttle protons and electrons from one bio-energy enzyme to another in a continuous cycle, thousands of times every second. Without enough coQ10 molecules, the cell's energy production system breaks down. A brain with a shortage of coQ10 is unable to function at top form, and may even degenerate faster over the years.

AN ELITE ANTIOXIDANT

CoQ10 does double duty—as the spark of cell energy—and a potent antioxidant. CoQ10 is a member of the elite force of five antioxidants that Dr. Packer elevates to the highest status in cell protection. CoQ10, along with vitamin E, works in the fatty parts of the cells where the potential for damage is worst. A key reason cells disintegrate, malfunction, and may be destroyed, is the huge assault on their fatty membranes, resulting in the most feared damage, called "lipid peroxidation." Such "lipid peroxidation" is the initial stage of the beginning of the end of a brain cell. If that toxic change can be avoided, your brain cells are much more likely to survive and generate needed energy. Another plus that makes coQ10 so powerful in brain cells: It not only fights lipid peroxidation, it also resuscitates vitamin E, a major force in shielding brain fats from peroxidation.

FIRST HEART, NOW BRAIN

For years, scientists concentrated on the danger of low coenzyme Q10 in heart cells, finding that the heart's energy slows down dramatically without enough coQ10, contributing to

THE MITOCHONDRIA MIRACLE

Each cell has thousands of mitochondria, where the complex chemistry that creates energy (read "life") occurs. All goes well if the mitochondria are normal. But through the years, these tiny structures are bombarded by free radicals, damaging their DNA, leaving them defective. How well a cell continues to generate energy depends on the proportion of normal mitochondria to defective ones, says Douglas Wallace, Ph.D., professor of biochemistry at Emory University. Accumulated DNA damage from aging can decrease the number of normal mitochondria to the point the cell becomes incapacitated, says Wallace. For example, defective mitochondria stop producing glutathione, a powerhouse antioxidant in brain cells. Most vulnerable are cells that require the most energy—namely in the brain and heart. What coenzyme Q10 does: facilitates the energy-generating process (electron transport) and scares off free radicals that render mitochondria defective.

The mitochondria of neurons need extra antioxidant protection because brain cells burn so much energy and are full of fat that must be detoxified if they are to function normally.

heart failure, and that restoring high levels could reenergize heart function. Only recently have scientists turned their attention to the malfunction of brain cells when coQ10 levels are low. As expected, the potential consequences of a disruption of energy production in brain cells due to a coQ10 shortage are every bit as serious as in heart cells. Obviously, since a brain without adequate coQ10 cannot work at full power, memory and learning abilities decline, and the brain appears to become more vulnerable to age-related neurodegenerative diseases, including Alzheimer's, Parkinson's, Huntington's, and ALS.

Unfortunately, aging robs the brain of coQ10; much less is produced internally as you get older, contributing to age-related brain disorders. At the same time, free radical activity revs up, making aging a double threat to neurons. Your once mighty mitochondria, young and vigorous, become tired and drained of energy as they age. One way to rejuvenate them: take coQ10.

CoQ10 MAKES BRAIN CELLS YOUNG AGAIN

CoQ10 is riding high among neuroscientists mainly due to an impressive series of studies by former Harvard neurologist Dr. M. Flint Beal, M.D., now chair of the neurology department at New York Hospital-Cornell Medical Center. Since it's known that coQ10 levels sink as you age, researchers needed to know whether a supplement of coQ10 would find its way to brain cells, replenishing them. Dr. Beal fed middle-aged lab animals high doses of coQ10. Autopsy examinations of their brain tissue showed that levels of coQ10 increased dramatically in the cerebral cortex of the animals. Moreover, coQ10 was most concentrated in the prime target, the brain mitochondria, where it's most needed. The longer the animals took coQ10, the higher the levels rose. Brain levels of coQ10 jumped 8 percent after one week, 16 percent after one month, and fully 30 percent after two months! This restored the levels of coQ10 to those seen in young animals. In other words, taking coQ10 dramatically rejuvenated brain cells. It's expected to have a similar effect on human brains.

CoQ10 Blocks ALS

In other striking experiments Dr. Beal's team found that coQ10 could increase the survival time of mice genetically bred to develop Lou Gehrig's disease (amyotrophic lateral sclerosis) and markedly block the development of brain injury characteristic of this disease. The brains of people with Lou Gehrig's typically form more free radicals and have abnormally low levels of antioxidants, along with lethargic mitochondria. It's the same situation you find in brains that are aging abnormally fast, says Dr. Packer.

Dr. Beal's intent: to see if coQ10 could save brain cells from ALS-type destruction. Injecting a specific poison, malonate, into the animals' brains typically destroys mitochondria, producing massive injury and death. He found that giving coQ10 along with the poison reduced the extent of the brain damage and prolonged the animals' lives. He found the same thing in the brains of animals genetically prone to a specific type brain damage found in Huntington's disease. CoQ10 virtually wiped out the occurrence of such brain injuries. It appears says Dr. Beal that coQ10 may be effective in combating various degenerative brain diseases, namely Alzheimer's, ALS, Parkinson's, and Huntington's.

Interestingly, taking coQ10 supplements pushed brain levels up in adult animals, but not in young ones. Presumably, younger animals already have brains saturated with coQ10. However, as you age, coQ10 levels decline, because your body makes less coQ10 and the rate of "lipid peroxidation" speeds up, using up coQ10 to fight off free radicals. The idea, then, to protect an aging brain from damage is to restore coQ10 levels to those of earlier days. In short, use coQ10 to rejuvenate your brain!

New Hope for Treating Parkinson's

CoQ10 looks extremely promising in preventing and treating Parkinson's disease, a degenerative brain disease. Scientists have discovered that Parkinson's involves two defects that coenzyme Q10 is good at fixing. One is a dysfunction in the mitochondria's energy production, the other, free radical damage to nerve cells that produce the neurotransmitter dopamine, located in a part of the brain called the substantia nigra. Researchers have also found that coenzyme Q10 is exceptionally low in people with Parkinson's. That clue led Dr. Beal and Cliff Shults, professor of neurosciences at the University of California, San Diego, to put coQ10 in the food of animals for a month before giving them, as well as control animals, a toxin designed to destroy dopamine-producing brain cells. It was exciting to note that coQ10-fed animals suffered much less brain damage and loss of dopamine than animals not given coQ10. This suggests that coQ10 could help prevent Parkinson's and/or retard its progression. High brain levels of coenzyme Q10 might ward off the demons that cripple dopamine production.

It was time to test the idea in humans. A preliminary study suggested that high doses of coenzyme Q10 (200 to 800 milligrams a day) stirred up dopamine-protecting activity in nerve cells. It was successful enough to prompt the National Institutes of Health to fund a full-scale double-blind investigation at twelve leading medical centers to see if coenzyme Q10 slows the worsening of Parkinson's. Patients not requiring medications such as Levodopa are taking doses of 600 or 1200 milligrams of coQ10 daily.

The National Institutes of Health has also launched a major trial of coQ10 in treating Huntington's disease—a genetic brain degenerative disease that affects up to 30,000 Americans. The test dose is also 600 milligrams or 1200 milligrams a day. Results of both studies are expected in 2001.

How Much?

There is no established brain dose of coQ10. Dr. Packer favors 30 milligrams a day, as does leading expert Dr. Denham Harman of the University of Nebraska. Other clinicians have suggested a daily antiaging dose of 5 to 10 milligrams. You may need more—100 to 200 milligrams— if you smoke, have heart disease, or a high risk of degenerative brain disease. Any supplement dose will greatly multiply what you get in food, which is typically one milligram of coQ10 daily, research shows. Unfortunately, coQ10 is expensive, because Japanese companies have a monopoly on its production.

Moreover, individuals vary greatly in how they absorb coQ10. Since coQ10 is fat-soluble, it's best to take it after you have eaten something, or along with a little fat, such as olive oil or peanut butter. The only way to determine whether you have low or high levels of coQ10 is to have a blood test. (See page 173.)

What type? CoQ10 is packaged under many brands. One reliable brand of coQ10 used in Dr. Beal's tests and in the new NIH clinical trials for Parkinson's is made by Vitaline Corporation, Ashland, Oregon. Mail order number: 800–648–4755.

Drugs Drive Down CoQ10

Taking anticholesterol drugs not only lowers your cholesterol, but also tends to deplete your reserves of coQ10, potentially leaving you with clean arteries but a dysfunctional brain. That's why if you are taking cholesterol-lowering drugs, called statins (prime examples are Mevacor and Zocor), you must be extra sure to take coQ10 supplements to preserve your brain as well as your heart.

> **BOTTOM LINE:** *If your brain cells are lethargic, it may be your fault for failing to give them enough coQ10. It can help immunize your brain against "normal" aging and even rejuvenate brains afflicted with neurodegenerative diseases.*

A WORD ABOUT A-CARNITINE AS BRAIN-BOOSTER

Another supplement that has energizing powers in brain cells is acetyl-L-carnitine, and some studies suggest your brain may get an added boost by taking a-carnitine along with coQ10. Such a-carnitine also pumps up energy production in the mitochondria of cells. Additionally, acetyl-L-carnitine helps retard the loss of receptors on brain cells and stimulates message transmission.

In tests, a-carnitine has improved the mental functioning of some people with Alzheimer's, but has not proved as effective as once hoped. Usual dose is 250 to 1000 milligrams a day. A reported side effect: vivid dreams. Don't take a-carnitine if you have epilepsy or manic depression (bipolar disorder). People with Alzheimer's should use it under a doctor's supervision.

Ginkgo:
A Boost for Aging Brains

It's the most promising well-tested nonprescription antiaging "smart drug" or "cognitive enhancer," say many researchers. It's ginkgo biloba, approved in Germany for a decade to revive failing memory. The scientific buzz on ginkgo is so good that countless prestigious American scientists and doctors, many in middle age, are now taking it, hoping to stave off memory loss as they get older. Dr. Jerry Cott, age fifty-two, chief of research on pharmacological treatment at the National Institute of Mental Health, takes 240 milligrams of ginkgo daily as "insurance" against declining memory. He thinks it's a reasonable and inexpensive precaution, based on current evidence. He also believes ginkgo has improved the mental functioning and well-being of his elderly mother who has Alzheimer's disease.

Dr. Norman Rosenthal, a research psychiatrist at NIMH, in his late forties, takes 120 milligrams of ginkgo every day. Dr. Lester Packer, age seventy, professor of cellular biology and chemistry at the University of California at Berkeley, takes 30 milligrams of ginkgo daily, as a brain-protecting antioxidant. Dr. Turin Itil, world-renowned neuropsychiatrist and author of pioneering studies on ginkgo and Alzheimer's disease, has been taking 120 milligrams of ginkgo daily for four years. In his seventies, he says it has made a remarkable difference, especially in recalling numbers. "Before I took ginkgo, I could never remember phone numbers. Now my secretary is amazed at how I can recall them. Practically all my friends and family over age sixty-five are taking ginkgo, at my suggestion," he adds. Dr. Itil is a clinical professor of psychiatry at New York University Medical Center and chairman of the World Health Organization's International Advisory Committee on the Diagnosis, Prevention, and Treatment of Alzheimer's Disease.

What do these prominent researchers know that you need to know? Why are they and thousands of other leading brain researchers and doctors throughout the world taking ginkgo biloba?

Compelling evidence is found in the pages of many medical journals worldwide. About 250 studies of ginkgo pharmacology and efficacy have been published in the last fifteen years. More than fifty controlled clinical trials, most done in Europe, proclaim ginkgo biloba a successful treatment for diminished age-related memory and concentration, increased absentmindness, confusion, dizziness, tinnitus (ringing in the ears), and Alzheimer's disease. Ginkgo is specifically approved by the German government for such conditions.

POWERFUL, DIVERSE PROTECTION

Ginkgo biloba, an extract from leaves of the ginkgo tree, promises so many brain-protecting properties it's impossible to know which are most important. Dr. Packer praises ginkgo's strong antioxidant activity. He has shown that ginkgo zaps two of the most virulent free radicals—superoxide and the hydroxyl radical—that readily savage brain cells. Dr. Packer also notes that ginkgo neutralizes the free radical nitric oxide that fosters blood vessel and brain cell damage, notably by triggering inflammation. Thus, ginkgo is an anti-inflammatory—a big plus for the brain.

Ginkgo increases circulation of blood and oxygen to the capillaries of the brain, studies show, probably by reducing blood viscosity. Many experts think this alone makes ginkgo a formidable brain-booster. Dr. Itil also notes that ginkgo increases glucose (sugar) metabolism in the brain which is another possible way ginkgo works to maintain or rejuvenate memory. French researchers found that ginkgo directly boosted neurotransmitter activity, possibly by restoring or preserving the integrity of nerve cell membranes.

Electroencephalograms (EEGs) show that ginkgo produces striking pharmacological activity in the brain. Dr. Itil found that in both young men, average age thirty-two, and elderly people with impaired memory, a standardized brand of ginkgo (Ginkgold) acted as a "cognitive activator," increasing alpha brain wave activity in all areas of the brain. The increased brain wave activity was evident within an hour to three hours after taking ginkgo. Gingko also may reverse brain aging by stimulating the regrowth of nerve cell receptors that have been lost to aging, and combating the process called "excitotoxicity" that disables and destroys brain cells.

GINKGO HELD OFF ALZHEIMER'S

Gingko's big moment came in 1997, in a double-blind study published in the *Journal of the American Medical Association*. Dr. Itil and colleagues, including Dr. Pierre Le Bars, tested ginkgo (known as Schwabe EGb761 or Ginkgold) in a daily dose of 120 milligrams on 137 patients with dementia caused either by strokes or Alzheimer's. After a year, fully 30 percent of those with dementia performed better on tests of memory and reasoning and were judged better in social behavior and mood by caregivers than those on placebo. Bottom line: Those on ginkgo did not show signs of worsening mental deterioration, as did those on the dummy pill, and even improved slightly in social functioning. Researchers speculated that a higher dose—240 milligrams daily—might be more effective when the brain deterioration is so advanced.

Many researchers start taking ginkgo soon after hitting middle age. Their rationale: If ginkgo retarded such a frightening disease as Alzheimer's, it makes sense that it can intervene earlier to prevent the symptoms of Alzheimer's in the first place. After all, as experts say, Alzheimer's does not come on overnight, but is a climactic event after years of gradual decline in brain functioning. Mild cognitive impairment (MCI), early signs of memory problems, is now thought to be a precursor of Alzheimer's disease. Thus, if you delay or prevent such early detrimental brain changes, you may never progress to dementia-type brain damage.

GINGKO GOES ON TRIAL

The National Institutes of Health is so convinced of the brain-saving potenial of ginkgo that it has initiated a first of its kind $15 million trial to see if the herb can halt memory deterioration and onset of dementia, including Alzheimers, in vulnerable individuals. "It's very exciting" says Dr. Cott. The double-blind study, conducted under the auspices of the National Center for Complementary and Alternative Medicine and the National Institute of Aging will give a daily dose of 240 milligrams of ginkgo or a placebo to 2,000 elderly men and women for six years. The subjects will also undergo tests of memory and general mental functioning. If those taking ginkgo are less apt to develop dementia or cognitive decline, researchers will have new proof of ginkgo's ability to deter or delay brain deterioration.

THE "PERFECT" PILL FOR NORMAL AGING

But far more important to most people is the ordinary erosion in mental function and memory that comes with age—

primarily a reduction in the speed of processing information and short-term memory needed to recall telephone numbers, names and faces, for example. Ginkgo seems ideally suited to deal with such age-related memory decline. As Dr. Pierre Le Bars, leading ginkgo researcher and assistant clinical professor at New York University, points out, "The evidence does not really show ginkgo to be an overall booster of memory as—for example, in expanding long-term storage and retrieval of information." Studies, he says, find that ginkgo primarily speeds up reaction times and accuracy involved in short-term and so-called "working memory" notably in people with some age-related decline.

In studies of sixty to sixty-five-year-olds with mild cognitive problems, ginkgo has improved short-term memory and working memory. Subjects were better able to focus on, store, and more rapidly retrieve recently learned information—such as a list of words—after taking ginkgo. That's why some say ginkgo fills the precise gap of mild memory deficits suffered during normal aging.

At what age does memory generally start to decline? In some people memory may grow worse at age thirty, but in others not until forty, fifty, sixty, or even later, says Dr. Itil. And for some, memory loss never progresses; in others, it declines rapidly. Dr. Itil warns that it's best to intervene immediately when you notice the first signs of memory impairment rather than waiting for it to worsen, possibly eventually progressing to dementia or Alzheimer's. The fact that so much brain cell damage in advanced years is now thought to stem from free-radical damage and low antioxidant defenses also makes antioxidant ginkgo look better than ever as a brain saver.

GINKGO VS. STROKES

Fascinating research at the National Institute on Aging suggests that taking ginkgo may cut the severity of brain damage after a stroke. In experiments, scientists gave gerbils ginkgo and then cut off blood flow to the brain, inducing a stroke. In such situations, the brain is hit with high concentrations of the toxic arachidonic acid that can cause extensive damage many ways, notably by releasing free radicals and producing inflammation. The longer the arachidonic acid stays around, the more brain cells it can damage. Thus, the brain tries to recycle it as quickly as possible. What gingko did in the gerbil brains is hasten the uptake or removal of arachidonic acid. In a similar gerbil study, ginkgo also blocked cell death in the hippocampus.

Extrapolated to humans, it suggests that providing brain cells with ginkgo ahead of time might save them from death and damage in case of stroke.

HOW MUCH?

Most early studies in Europe used a standard dose of 120 milligrams of ginkgo daily. Some researchers now advocate higher doses—240 milligrams daily. Even doses as high as 600 milligrams have been used experimentally. Still, the lower dose of 120 milligrams may, in fact, be best for most older people with the beginnings of memory problems. An interesting 1998 Danish study showed that 120 milligrams of ginkgo significantly improved intellectual function in men and women, average age seventy-four, with mild to moderate cognitive impairment. But a double daily dose of 240 milligrams, surprisingly, did not!

Those on the lower 120 milligram ginkgo dose scored higher on tests of attention, concentration, and short-term verbal memory after three months. Their diastolic blood pressure also went down. But those taking the higher 240 milligram dose did not improve test scores. Moreover, those on the high dose reported side effects, including sleep disturbances, dizziness, and dyspepsia.

It's possible that ginkgo may have an "optimal" dose range for some people, beyond which too little or too much is not beneficial. Dr. Le Bars suggests first trying 120 milligrams and raising it after three to six months if you sense no improvement. Research shows you should notice improvement, he says, after a month or so. If you "don't feel better" after four to six weeks of taking 120 milligrams, you can bump it up to 240 milligrams, but if that brings no signs of improvement in a few months, "forget it," advises Dr. Le Bars. "You, along with half of the population, are not a ginkgo responder."

Dr. Le Bars notes that not everyone can expect to get an intellectual boost from ginkgo. Only 50 percent at most of those who take ginkgo see improvement, research shows. Among those with severe memory loss or Alzheimer's the figure is lower—30 to 40 percent. Any ginkgo benefit stops with 50 percent of the population, for unknown reasons, even at the higher dose of 240 milligrams daily, concludes Dr. Le Bars. He also feels that ginkgo is more apt to forestall early memory decline than to slow down or reverse advanced dysfunction, as in Alzheimer's.

How Safe?

Ginkgo has been heralded as very safe, inducing only minor and reversible side effects, such as nausea. Recently, a couple of cases of excessive bleeding have been reported after taking ginkgo. Whether ginkgo was a contributing cause is unknown. However, some experts now advise anyone with a known bleeding problem, a history of hemorrhagic stroke, or who is regularly taking anticoagulants such as Coumadin or aspirin for heart disease, to consult a doctor before taking ginkgo. "It's possible ginkgo might contribute to a bleeding problem," says Dr. Le Bars, "although the chances are very remote." Still, such a hazard can be avoided by having your doctor check the coagulation factors of your blood. If you are not on regular blood thinners, including aspirin, there should be no danger, says Dr. Le Bars.

What type? Not all ginkgo on the market is equal. Tests have found that even reputably "standardized" brands do not have equal benefits on the brain. In a test of three such commercial ginkgo products by Dr. Itil, only one EGb 761 (sold as Ginkgold) performed as a "cognitive enhancer."

A WORD ABOUT PYCNOGENOL™

Although ginkgo has been more widely tested as a brain-booster, some experts say another natural extract made from pine bark has extraordinary potential in protecting the brain from age-related deterioration and mental decline. It is Pycnogenol™, a strong antioxidant supplement produced in France and distributed by the Henkel Company in the United States.

New evidence from the Berkeley laboratory of Dr. Lester Packer shows that Pycnogenol possesses strong powers against certain free radicals, including nitric oxide that can be toxic to brain cells, especially in brains vulnerable to Alzheimer's, Parkinson's and other neurodegenerative diseases. Dr. Packer predicts that as new research reveals the brain-protective powers of Pycnogenol, it, like ginkgo, will become widely popular as a brain-boosting supplement.

BOTTOM LINE: *Taking ginkgo may slow down brain damage such as Alzheimer's that causes intellectual decay, and may help correct some memory lapses and cognitive impairment due to normal aging. There's no evidence ginkgo is a "smart drug" in the sense of sharpening memory or boosting mental powers beyond normal functioning. It is not a pill young people could count on to boost scores on a test, for example. Indeed, gingko's essence seems to be in slowing the gradual decline in mental faculties, notably in aging brains, because of its diverse pharmacological activity, including its strong antioxidant properties.*

Phosphatidylserine (PS): Memory Rejuvenator

One of the most scientifically promising memory enhancers is a substance with the tongue-twisting name phosphatidylserine (*fos'fuh tid'ill ser een*). Most experts simply call it PS. It's a fatty nutrient present in all cell membranes, but most concentrated in brain cells. It has no trouble zipping through the blood-brain barrier. It gets to the brain within minutes after it's absorbed. This is very good news for those whose brains need more PS. And that is about everybody over age forty.

> *"I've tested close to a hundred compounds for their effects on human memory, and phosphatidylserine (PS) is the most impressive one I've found so far."*
> —Thomas Crook, former chief of the Geriatric Psychopharmacology Program at the National Institute of Mental Health and author of *The Memory Cure*

PS is one of the few nonprescription memory boosters that commands respect from hard-core brain investigators, because numerous studies, most done in the early 1990s, indicate it can rejuvenate memory. Reportedly, more than twenty-five human studies, about half of them double-blind—the "gold standard" for testing—have found phosphatidylserine effective in revving up failing memory.

PS's most credentialed champion is an authority on memory loss, Thomas H. Crook III, Ph.D. For fourteen years he was a research psychologist at the prestigious National Institute of Mental Health. As president of Psychologix, Inc., a research organization in Scottsdale, Arizona, he now conducts private research for pharmaceutical companies. It was Dr. Crook's 1991 study that propelled phosphatidylserine to scientific notice. PS at the time was considered a prescription drug; it was later reclassified as an over-the-counter "dietary supplement." In collaboration with researchers at Vanderbilt University School of Medicine and Stanford University, Dr. Crook studied the memory effects of PS on 149 persons, ages fifty to seventy-five. All had typical age-related memory impairment. Initially, the investigators were "extremely skeptical," because they knew of no substance that could delay age-related memory loss, let alone reverse it. They soon decided PS was unique.

ERASES MEMORY DECLINE

For twelve weeks, half of the subjects took 100 milligrams of PS three times a day at mealtimes. The others took an inactive look-alike "sugar pill" or placebo. All subjects took a battery of neuropsychological tests at the start of the study and at three-week intervals. By the end of the study it was clear that those taking PS scored about 30 percent higher on tests of memory and learning. Further, PS takers with the worst memory deficits benefited the most. They were better at remembering names, faces, telephone numbers, and recalling paragraphs; their concentration also improved. The investigators concluded that PS shaved twelve years off the normal expected decline in specific aspects of memory performance! In short, if a person's "cognitive age" for remembering faces was equivalent to age sixty-four, PS reversed it to age fifty-two—a year's rollback for each week of taking the supplement. Further, the memory hike persisted for a month after subjects stopped taking PS.

"PS is not a magic bullet," says Dr. Crook. "It's not like

you're seventy-five and take it and you become twenty-five. But it is the first thing we've ever seen of many, many compounds that does have a clear measurable effect—and that effect is about twelve years of rolling back the clock. I really firmly believe that PS can roll back virtually all age-related memory impairment."

Extensive foreign research supports Dr. Crook's findings. Since the early 1980s, Italian investigators have used PS widely to revitalize memory in older persons. One of the most impressive double-blind studies was done in 1987 by researchers at Italy's University of Catania. For three months 170 patients with moderately impaired cognitive function took either a daily PS dose of 300 milligrams or a placebo. Those getting PS surpassed the placebo group on neuropsychological tests measuring cognitive function, including memory. In two memory measures—semantic association ability and verbal fluency—PS takers scored 50 percent higher than placebo takers.

The largest double-blind Italian study of 425 older persons with moderate to severe intellectual decline showed that PS (300 milligrams daily for six months) improved scores on tests of total recall, long-term memory storage, and long-term retrieval of learned information. PS also bolstered communication and social interaction and lessened apathy and withdrawal.

"As laboratory rats reach middle age, they are less able to negotiate mazes. If they take PS, they stay smart into old age."
—Parris M. Kidd, Ph.D., authority on PS, consultant for Lucas Meyer, makers of PS

What about Alzheimer's disease? Not surprisingly, PS has been tested on people with dementia and Alzheimer's. It may help in some cases, but overall, it has not proved as effective in treating Alzheimer's, especially in the advanced stages, as in rejuvenating memory in ordinary people without the disease. For example, in 1992 Dr. Crook and colleagues at Vanderbilt University gave PS to patients with Alzheimer's; they concluded it did boost cognitive functioning in the early stages of the disease. But in those with more advanced Alzheimer's any PS-induced cognitive improvements were extremely modest and subtle.

Dr. Crook calls PS an ideal "memory cure" for the precise type memory decline that is typical after middle age. It's unlikely PS will cure Alzheimer's. Nor will it give you a super memory you never had before. But it may help restore the memory you would have had if normal aging had not eroded it.

BOTTOM LINE: *PS may slow, stop, or restore memory losses due to normal aging.*

SOYBEAN PS—BETTER YET

Before the "mad cow disease" scare, PS supplements were derived from cow brains, and most early studies were done with this so-called bovine PS. Today, PS is derived from soybeans entirely, and about 95 percent of it sold as a supplement is made by one company, Lucas Meyer in Decatur, Illinois, under the trademark Leci-PS. It is then packaged by a hundred or so individual companies and sold under many different brands. Since much of the evidence for PS effectiveness came from animal-type PS, the question arises: Is the current PS made from plants—soybeans—equally effective?

Dr. Crook proclaims soy-type PS supplements identical in memory-boosting powers, even superior in some aspects, to the formerly used bovine PS. A recent double-blind test was an endorsement of soy Leci-PS. Dr. Crook found that people with memory troubles who took 300 milligrams a day of soybean PS (Leci PS™) for twelve weeks demonstrated striking improvement: Compared with placebo-takers, their ability to learn and remember written information jumped 33 percent; remembering names immediately after an introduction skyrocketed 24 percent; recalling names one hour after introduction rose 33 percent over the placebo group.

Here's what that means in years of memory rejuvenation. Dr. Crook figures that taking soy PS rolled back the clock fourteen years in remembering names after introduction, twelve years in learning and recalling written information, seven years in recognizing someone previously seen, and four years in dialing a ten-digit telephone number from memory—all within three months.

How does PS work? It basically energizes or revs up the brain. Proof positive of PS's global impact on brain performance comes from PET scans and electroencephalogram (EEG) readings. Even in young men, injecting phosphatidylserine intravenously boosted alpha brain rhythms an average 15 to 20 percent, as shown on EEGs; such alpha activity is typically lower in aged and cognitively impaired brains.

In older subjects with mild memory problems oral doses of PS (300 milligrams daily) boosted sagging EEG "power" values to almost normal; scores on cognitive tests went up accordingly.

Most remarkable, German neurologists at the Max Planck Institute in Cologne did PET scans before and after giving 500 milligrams a day of PS for three weeks to patients with probable Alzheimer's disease. While subjects took a mental test, PET scans recorded an increased "activation" of the brain. Before PS, the brain images were a calm sea of blue with only a few tiny dots of yellow and red, signifying low levels of glucose metabolism and brain activity. After PS treatment, the brain images are ablaze with large bright yellow patches and red dots, clearly illustrating a huge jump in activity and glucose metabolism in various regions of the brain. The greater brain activity induced by PS corresponded with higher scores on tests of cognitive functioning.

It is thought that the brain's increased energy comes because PS enhances message transmission in nerve cells. Studies show PS raises levels of some neurotransmitters, particularly the memory-booster acetylcholine and dopamine; it also speeds up conduction of nerve impulses and modifies the structure and fatty consistency of neuron membranes and receptors, making neurotransmitters more efficient, thus facilitating cell to cell communication. PS also helps block the erosion of dendrite connections that normally occurs during aging. And it even helps protect cell membranes from free-radical damage.

What's the right dose? The standard dose in tests is a 100 milligram pill taken three times a day (at mealtimes) for a total daily dose of 300 milligrams. That's what Dr. Crook, age fifty-five, takes to protect his memory from age-related decline, and recommends for at least the first month. After that you can drop to one 100-milligram pill per day, or you can continue at 300 milligrams per day. Unfortunately, PS is expensive, about $1 per 100-milligram pill, which adds up to $90 per month for the high dose. An alternative: Start and continue with just 100 milligrams per day, if that is more affordable. The difference, says Dr. Crook: You should see improvement on the higher 300 milligram dose after three or four weeks. The lower 100 milligram dose may take eight or ten weeks to produce a memory boost.

What type PS? PS is widely available in health food stores, drugstores, and some supermarkets. It comes in either gel capsule or pill and is packaged under more than 100 different brands. Look for the trademark Leci-PS on the label or package; this assures you it contains the right stuff. Analyses of PS from other manufacturers have revealed poor quality and impurities. Fortunately, since almost all the soy PS made is Leci-PS™, it's hard to go wrong, and it's okay to buy the least expensive brand. Packagers sell it for varying prices.

How safe is it? PS's safety record is impressive. Although millions of Italians have taken PS for twenty years, there are no reports of significant side effects or even of interactions with pharmaceutical drugs. However, PS authority Dr. Parris Kidd cautions that in rare cases, downing high doses—200 milligrams or more of PS at one time—might cause nausea. To avoid this possibility, take PS with meals, he advises. Taking it just before going to bed might delay your falling asleep, Dr. Kidd adds.

What about food? You eat small amounts of PS in fish, soy foods, rice, and green leafy vegetables. But it's probably not enough to protect your memory from the wounds of aging after middle age.

Choline:
The Brain's Memory Architect

Choline, an amino acid, may protect the brain throughout life—from the womb to very old age. Indeed, if your mother eats enough choline to satiate your fetal brain, you may enjoy a lifetime of superior intellect and not even have to worry about a declining memory as you get old. That's a remarkable new finding from laboratory animals, that researchers say may translate to humans, although such human studies have not been done.

What researchers have found is phenomenal: That giving rats choline halfway through pregnancy makes a permanent mark on the fetal brain—dictating how its cells organize to mold and wire the brain, essentially building in an "excess memory capacity" that endures throughout life. In a series of experiments, scientists at Duke University Medical Center fed pregnant rats normal choline, extra choline, or no choline and then studied the mental functioning and brains of their offspring.

Clearly, the rats that got the extra choline in the womb had vastly superior brains; as infants and adults they displayed better memory and learning capabilities. Indeed, postmortem examinations revealed superbly efficient brain circuits for transmitting messages. The neurons in their hippocampus, the brain's memory processing center, responded instantly to the tiniest electrical probe, indicating their brains were primed to learn rapidly. Awesome as it seems, the extra infusion of a single nutrient, choline, enabled nature to assemble a brain of extraordinary quality.

On the other hand, rats deprived of choline in utero had sluggish brains and impaired memory when they grew up.

AN ANTIDOTE TO MEMORY LOSS
Even more startling, as the high-choline offspring entered old age, their brain function remained undiminished. Their memory did not fade, as it did in rats not given choline prenatally. In very old age, choline-primed rats made only half as many memory errors when searching through mazes for food as did geriatric rats whose pregnant mothers had not been given extra choline.

> *"The ramifications of this could be profound. We've found that manipulating one single nutrient for a few days during gestation has a lifelong effect on how brains function. In theory, we could develop ways to significantly reduce age-related memory deficits."*—Dr. Scott Swartzwelder, neuropsychologist, Duke University

How could choline received before birth possibly be so powerful and long-lasting as to prevent memory deterioration in old age? Researchers speculate that choline might slow down the entire aging process, the brain included. Or, more probable, choline helps construct a brain with such a superior anatomical network of neurons and connections—a large reserve of brain power and efficient memory processing—that age-related erosion is insignificant to memory functioning later in life.

Choline does dramatically change the very structure of memory centers in the hippocampus and septum of the developing fetal brain, declares Dr. Steven Zeisel, M.D., a world expert on choline, and chairman of nutrition at the University of North Carolina School of Medicine at Chapel Hill. Dr. Zeisel and colleagues found that when choline is lacking, cell division in the fetal brain is reduced, cells migrate abnormally, and increasing numbers of brain cells die prematurely. "For the first time, we have shown that the very structure of the brain is influenced by what mothers eat during pregnancy. Mainly, the specific nutrient choline appears to be critical."

A SECOND CHANCE

But what if your mother failed to give your fetal brain lots of choline? Will eating choline later as a child, adult, or in old age improve your mental functioning? It's a good bet, say experts, although you cannot count on choline to completely reorganize the way your brain circuits work. Still, birth does not put an end to the brain's need for choline.

Choline is particularly essential for infants, whose brains are still developing. So if a mother missed providing lots of choline in the womb, there is a second chance. Not surprisingly, breast milk, also depending on a mother's diet, is very rich in choline, which is one more brain-boosting reason to breast-feed. Infant formulas made from both cow's milk and soy are required to add choline, but they do not contain as much as human breast milk.

Breast-feeding is definitely preferred, and may make a difference in your baby's brain. "Because infant formulas vary so much from human breast milk," says Dr. Zeisel, "it's not unreasonable to worry that some differences in intellectual performance that we see could be due to changes in the availability of choline in utero and shortly after birth in some kids."

Besides building strong brains, choline is also vital in keeping brain cells functioning throughout life. For one thing, choline is a precursor (building block) for acetylcholine, the neurotransmitter vital to encoding memory.

When choline is in good supply, your neurons are more apt to make and release acetylcholine. Blocking production of acetylcholine in brain cells impairs memory; flooding brain cells with acetylcholine may overcome some memory deficits. That's the theory of some drugs used to treat Alzheimer's and dementia. Choline is a critical constituent of fat in brain cell membranes, influencing their structure and facilitating transmission of signals from the cell exterior to the nucleus, a momentous task. Additionally, choline

---

FIVE WAYS CHOLINE BUILDS BETTER BRAINS

- Choline is the raw material for synthesis of acetylcholine, the memory neurotransmitter with widespread and diverse activity in brain cells.
- Choline combined with fatty acids to make choline-phospholipids gives structure to cell membranes, and helps regulate transmission of signals between the cell exterior and the nucleus, a mighty influence in brain cell business.
- Choline added to drinking water spurred growth of new dendritic spines in the cerebral cortexes of old mice. Their memory and learning improved, too.
- Choline helps break down homocysteine, a brain toxin.
- Choline in fetal brains helps dictate the very architecture and wiring, and thus the intellectual capacity of the brain after birth and into old age.

helps suppress homocysteine in the blood that is associated with brain disturbances, memory damage, and even Alzheimer's, and strokes.

According to extensive research, choline improves memory and learning in many species, including rats, mice, mollusks, and humans. Of course, tests in laboratory animals do not prove that humans build brains the same way. But decades of research have been eerily accurate in making the leap from what happens in the brains of small mammals to how the human brain works. It's probable that if scientists discover a brain secret in other mammals, it will eventually be confirmed in humans. Growing new brain cells is a prime case in point: Thirty years before it was detected in humans, scientists had demonstrated it in laboratory animals.

It's unclear to what extent taking supplemental choline later in life may boost human memory or intellectual performance. Some studies find benefits; others do not. One recent experiment with eighty college students found improvement on tests of explicit memory in those who took 25 grams of lecithin that supplied 3750 milligrams of choline. There was no memory benefit from taking just ten grams of lecithin. Specifically, the students were better able to memorize a series of nonsense syllables about an hour and a half after taking the choline. Interestingly, the memory boost was greatest in "slow learners," leading researchers to suspect that the slow learners had subnormal levels of choline to begin with. Thus, a supplement corrected a slight deficiency.

This may mean, they said, that choline works best to improve memory in slow learners and the elderly who may have abnormally low choline. The double-blind controlled study was conducted by psychologists at several California universities, including Stanford.

Choline has boosted memory in older adults. Florence Safford, D.S.W., of Florida International University, had forty-one healthy people, ages fifty through eighty, take 500 milligrams of choline (found in two tablespoons of lecithin granules) every day for five weeks. She says they reported diminished memory lapses, such as forgetting names, misplacing items, remembering names on the tip of their tongue. Indeed, their memory lapses were about half those of comparable subjects not getting choline-lecithin—down from an average 35 lapses per week to 19 per week.

However, other more rigorous double-blind studies have not found mental benefits in adults taking choline. One explanation: The choline in food or supplements that gets into your bloodstream may not make it into your brain. Around middle age, the ability to transport choline from the blood to the brain tends to decline, say brain experts.

Regardless of whether high doses of choline hypes memory in adults, everybody still needs choline in the diet or through supplements for optimal brain functioning. Experts now consider choline an essential or required nutrient for all ages. Your body cannot make enough choline for optimum health.

> **BRAIN ALERT:** *Choline has become a slowly vanishing nutrient as Americans switched to very low fat diets and denounced eggs, one of the richest sources of choline.*

EGGS AS BRAIN FOOD

You may be surprised to learn that egg yolks are one of the highest and most reliable sources of choline. Thus, avoiding or severely restricting eggs may be harmful to brain functioning. The consumption of eggs has plummeted in the last thirty years due to warnings that the yolk is high in artery-clogging cholesterol. Consequently, intake of choline dropped sharply, since egg yolk is a major source of choline. Now, much new evidence shows that the amount of cholesterol in food is not a primary cause of raising cholesterol in the blood. High cholesterol is caused mainly by eating saturated fats, as in milk, butter, cheese, and meat.

Indeed, the egg is being exonerated. In April 1999, Harvard researchers proclaimed that an egg a day is unlikely to increase the risk of heart disease or strokes, according to a new analysis of the Harvard Nurses' Health Study and the Health Professionals Follow Up Study. Research tracked the egg consumption of 100,000 people for more than a decade. Harvard's Frank B. Hu, M.D., and colleagues, concluded that a daily egg is not harmful—and may even help prevent heart disease, because eggs contain nutrients, including antioxidants, folic acid, other B vitamins, and unsaturated fat that may counteract any ill effect from the yolk's high cholesterol. Another one of those beneficial nutrients is choline.

How Much Choline Do You Need Daily?

Adult men	550 mg	
Adult women	425 mg	
Pregnant women		450 mg
Lactating women		550 mg

How Much Is Too Much?

Upper tolerable upper daily intake for:

Children	1000 mg
Adults	3500 mg

SOURCE: National Academy of Sciences.

WHERE TO FIND CHOLINE

Best food sources: Egg yolks, peanuts, wheat germ, liver, meat, fish, milk, cheese, vegetables—mainly broccoli, cabbage, and cauliflower.

What about supplements? If you want to take choline supplements, the best bet is lecithin rather than straight choline. High doses of pure choline leave you smelling "fishy," say experts. Lecithin, which is 20 percent choline, is a far better source. Lecithin comes in various forms (the scientific name is phosphatidylcholine), including granules that you can dissolve in a liquid, such as juice or milk, or sprinkle on cereal. A tablespoon of lecithin granules supplies about 250 milligrams of choline.

Lecithin supplements appear very safe, even at high doses, according to government tests.

Huperzine:
Promising Alzheimer's Drug

An herbal supplement on the fast track for scientific recognition as a treatment for Alzheimer's is Huperzine A, a plant extract derived from Chinese club moss. Evidence that it may revitalize memory and help improve focus and concentration is causing a stir among top scientists, including research psychiatrists at the National Institute of Mental Health and academic pharmacologists. Debasis Bagchi, Ph.D., associate professor at Creighton University School of Pharmacy, says Huperzine A holds great promise "for a wide range of memory and brain disorders, including Alzheimer's disease."

Huperzine has been used for centuries in Chinese folk medicine to rejuvenate memory in older people.

The "memory moss" is said to work much like prescription drugs now approved for treating Alzheimer's. The key to both Huperzine A and such drugs is manipulation of the brain transmitter acetylcholine, known as the "memory molecule." Acetylcholine is abnormally low in Alzheimer' brains, because damaged nerve cells no longer synthesize it and an enzyme (acetylcholinesterase) keeps breaking down and whisking away what little is made. Huperzine A, like other memory-preserving drugs, is believed to block the enzyme from destroying acetylcholine, thus preserving more to facilitate transmission of electrical impulses between neurons. Technically, Huperzine A, like the approved Alzheimer's drugs, is called an "acetylcholinesterase inhibitor."

Many studies, most done in China, show that Huperzine surpassed the two major approved pharmaceutical drugs for Alzheimer's disease, Aricept (donepezil) and Cognex (tacrine), in reversing memory deficits in aging animals. Huperzine's activity is also reportedly long-lasting. One test in young healthy volunteers showed that Huperzine A blocked the target enzyme for 288 minutes, allowing more acetylcholine to circulate in the brain, whereas the prescription drug physotigmine inhibited the enzyme for only twenty minutes.

A recent double-blind trial at Zhejiang Medical University in Shanghai tested Huperzine on Alzheimer's patients. Half got the real thing, half a placebo for two months. Mental cognition was measured by "gold standard" tests, including the Wechsler Memory Scale and the Mini-Mental State Examination scale. Those getting Huperzine did 36 percent better than those on placebo.

Huperzine also reportedly improved mental function in patients with multi-infarct dementia, caused by repeated mini-strokes, as well as victims of myasthenia gravis, a neuromuscular disease.

What makes Huperzine so attractive is its apparent lack of serious side effects and very low toxicity, a big plus, since approved prescription drugs with the same mechanism of action inflict brutal side effects, notably liver toxicity. Some government authorities, however, are concerned that Huperzine, a drug reportedly as potent as current prescription drugs, can be sold to treat Alzheimer's without prescription, without FDA approval and without undergoing clinical trials in the United States. They think, at the very least, it should be used only with a doctor's supervision.

However, Alan P. Kozikowski, director of the Drug Discovery Program at Georgetown Medical Center in Washington, D.C., who first synthesized Huperzine, says its use is not limited to those with Alzheimer's, but benefits anyone worried about memory loss. "Anyone who is feeling some problem with memory recall will probably want it," he has said. "I've tried it myself. It does make you feel more alert."

How much? The typical dosage that benefited Alzheimer's patients in Chinese studies is 200 micrograms twice a day. But much less may also work. Alan Mazurek, M.D., a neurologist in private practice in Rockville Center, New York, recently reported that half of a small group of Alzheimer's patients improved in mental function after they took 100 micrograms of Huperzine A a day.

Despite Huperzine's promising track record, the argument that it equals efficacy of current drugs may not be a sterling recommendation. New findings published in the *Journal of the American Medical Association* claim that current prescription drugs, designed to preserve acetylcholine, are effective only in patients with *advanced* Alzheimer's, not in milder cases. If so, Huperzine might be of little or no benefit to people with mild to moderate memory disorders. More clinical trials are needed—and some are underway—to determine the memory boosting potential of Huperzine A. In the meantime, herbal authority California physician Ray Sahelian, author of numerous well-respected books on herbal remedies, advises using Huperzine A only as a treatment for Alzheimer's and not as a way to try to boost normal memory.

St. John's Wort:
Natural Prozac

If you are depressed, a pill made from the plant St. John's wort may boost your mood. St. John's wort, also called hypericum, is now widely accepted by doctors in this country for relieving mild to moderate depression after having been used successfully for decades in Europe, notably Germany. There is no question it works, says Norman Rosenthal, M.D., senior research psychiatrist at the National Institute of Mental Health and author of the book *St. John's Wort: The Herbal Way to Feeling Good*. In fact, many doctors now see St. John's wort as the first "drug" to try before conventional prescription antidepressants, such as Prozac and Zoloft. Such strong pharmaceutical drugs often have serious side effects, in contrast with St. John's wort which has only minimal adverse effects.

Worldwide, St. John's wort is the most commonly used antidepressant. More than seven million Americans now take it.

St. John's wort has proved to be an effective antidepressant in numerous double-blind studies in Europe. One analysis of many studies showed that St. John's wort relieved symptoms of mild to moderate depression partially or totally in 80 percent of about 3250 patients. It can work as well or better than prescription drugs, or in some cases along with prescription drugs.

The evidence for St. John's wort is so impressive that the National Institutes of Health has launched a major two-year study of effectiveness of the herb in treating mild to moderate depression at twelve U.S. medical centers, coordinated by Duke University. The brand used in the study: an extensively tested German product made by Lichtwer Pharma (LI160 or Jarsin) and sold under the name Kira in the United States. It is available over the counter without prescription.

Here are the types of depression that call for trying St. John's wort, according to Dr. Rosenthal: mild depression; short-term stress associated with depression and anxiety; moderate depression; depression in those who are very sensitive to, or concerned about, side effects; winter depression (seasonal affective disorder, or SAD); depression in the elderly; dysthymia (chronic low grade unhappiness).

New research shows that St. John's wort is especially good in treating the "winter blues," known as seasonal affective disorder (SAD) that comes with the dark days of winter. British investigators compared St. John's wort with light box therapy, which is known to be very successful in relieving SAD. St. John's wort was virtually as effective as light therapy after eight weeks. Among 301 Britons suffering from SAD, half were randomized to use the light box, the other half got St. John's wort. The severity of SAD symptoms, including depression, sleep disturbance, and lethargy, decreased 39 percent in those taking St. John's wort and 43 percent in those using the light box therapy, which was not a significant difference, said researchers. Of course, taking a pill is less hassle than using a light box, they pointed out.

It is not totally clear how St. John's wort relieves depression. Initially, researchers believed it worked the same way as so-called selective serotonin reuptake inhibitors (SSRIs) that include Prozac. The herb's main ingredient, hypericin, supposedly manipulated the neurotransmitter serotonin which helps govern mood. But now experts think St. John's wort affects other neurotransmitters as well, and other chemicals in the remedy also appear active. Most likely, many ingredients in St. John's wort work together for a total benefit unlike that found in synthetic antidepressants.

Recommended dose: a daily total of 900 milligrams taken in doses of 300 milligrams three times a day. Although some people may get relief with one or two tablets, others require more than three tablets.

Depression may lift within a few days of starting St. John's wort, or the full effect may take six weeks. Generally, however, you should see some improvement after three weeks of taking 900 milligrams daily, says Dr. Rosenthal. If you don't, you may want to increase the dose, or consider a conventional antidepressant in lieu of or in addition to St. John's wort. Be sure to consult a doctor.

Potential side effects: Most common are minor side effects such as gastrointestinal irritation, nausea, indigestion, abdominal pains. Studies show such side effects to be very low—about $2^{1}/_{2}$ percent. Exposure to sunlight if taking St. John's wort could be hazardous. One woman on St. John's wort experienced temporary nerve damage causing painful sensitivity in areas of the body exposed to the sun, according to a recent report in the medical journal *Lancet*. Symptoms disappeared after the woman stopped taking the herb.

Restrict alcohol to no more than a glass or two of beer or wine or one mixed drink when you are taking St. John's wort.

Cautions: Don't substitute St. John's wort for prescription antidepressants without first consulting your doctor. Don't take St. John's wort along with prescription antidepressants; the two could produce a hazardous interaction. Do not self-diagnose depression: Your symptoms could come from another medical cause; see a health professional. Don't take St. John's wort if you are pregnant. If you have bipolar, manic depression, use St. John's wort only under the close supervision of a doctor. It may or may not work.

Further, St. John's wort is designed to treat people with clinical signs of mild to moderate depression, and does not work as a casual "upper" for people who are just temporarily feeling down. Nor is there convincing evidence that it relieves severe depression.

Consumer advice: Some laboratory analyses of St. John's wort have found exceptionally low levels of the reputed active ingredient in some brands. One test in 1999 detected only 5 percent of the amount of active ingredient claimed on the label of one product. Varro Tyler, dean emeritus of Purdue University's School of Pharmacy and a leading authority on herbal remedies, advises always buying St. John's wort that is "standardized" to contain .3 percent of hypericin. Even then you can't be sure.

Your most reliable bet: Kira, which is the brand used in many studies, including the new one sponsored by the National Institutes of Health.

"SAMMY":
The New Antidepressant

A few years ago St. John's wort shot to fame as the natural depression cure of choice—the preferred alternative to prescription antidepressants. Now comes a pill called SAM-e ("Sammy") or S-adenosyl-methionine with rival powers. "It's the best antidepressant I've ever prescribed," says psychiatrist Richard Brown at Columbia University College of Physicians and Surgeons, and coauthor of a new book on SAM-e, *Stop Depression Now*.

Like St. John's wort, SAM-e hails from Europe, where it has been used for two decades to relieve depression, as well as osteoarthritis. Extensive research (about forty studies, most done in Europe) indicates that SAM-e combats depression as well as or sometimes better than state-of-the-art pharmaceuticals. Generally, controlled studies claim that SAM-e has a 70 percent success rate, about the same as conventional drug therapy. But SAM-e works faster and without troubling side effects, making it unique and preferable, say advocates.

Indeed, the first double-blind study of SAM-e by Italian researchers on severely depressed patients found that 100 percent of them improved on the supplement. A few almost completely recovered within four days. A major 1994 Italian review of two decades of studies (a meta-analysis) involving more than 1000 patients showed that SAM-e always relieved depression better than a placebo and always at least matched the effectiveness of tricyclic antidepressants. In some cases, SAM-e surpassed prescription drugs.

Researchers at the University of California at Irvine, for example, pitted SAM-e against desipramine, a tricyclic antidepressant, in a test of twenty-six depressed patients. Sixty-two percent of patients taking SAM-e improved compared with 50 percent taking desipramine.

SAM-e is something you make yourself. It is a natural constituent of cells, synthesized in the body from the essential amino acid L-methionine and ATP, the cellular energy chemical. SAM-e is a star player in the cell's energy production. Encouraged by folic acid and vitamin B_{12}, SAM-e donates a bit of itself (methyl group) to nearby cells, which is "an important event at the molecular level," as one scientist says. This crucial methyl transfer stimulates thirty-five vital chemical reactions in cells with widespread effects. Among other things, it promotes fluidity of cell membranes—a big thing in nerve cell functions—and production of good-mood neurotransmitters, mainly serotonin and dopamine. It's thought that stimulating serotonin and dopamine is a prime way SAM-e fights depression. When depressed people take SAM-e, there's evidence of increased serotonin and dopamine in their nervous systems.

SAM-e performs another miracle in your brain. Nerve cells must have SAM-e as raw material to synthesize glutathione, the main heavyweight antioxidant in neutralizing specific brain toxins and neuron-mutilating free radicals. Glutathione also has brain-protecting anti-inflammatory properties. Guaranteeing cells enough SAM-e to produce glutathione may be reason enough to take the supplement. Brain levels of both glutathione and SAM-e decline as we age. Oddly, taking glutathione supplements does not increase cellular or blood levels of the substance. But taking

SAM-e does, making it one of the few reliable ways of boosting precious glutathione.

There's also some evidence, says Teodoro Bottiglieri, Ph.D, director of neuropharmacology at Baylor University Medical Center in Dallas, that SAM-e may benefit people with dementia, including Alzheimer's. Dr. Bottiglieri, who has studied SAM-e for nearly twenty years, found abnormally low levels of SAM-e in the cerebrospinal fluid of Alzheimer's patients.

> *"The nicest thing about SAM-e is it works as well as standard prescription medications, but it has fewer side effects and it works faster, so people feel better sooner."*—Dr. Richard Brown, Columbia University

QUICK RELIEF

One of the great attractions of SAM-e is how rapidly it can bring relief. Conventional antidepressants usually take four to six weeks to elevate mood. Depression lifts in patients taking SAM-e sometimes within days. In a double-blind trial of depressed postmenopausal women, Italian researchers noted that SAM-e (in high daily doses of 1600 milligrams) relieved depression after ten days. Dr. Maurizio Fava, director of the Depression Clinic and Research Program at Massachusetts General Hospital in Boston, found that injecting patients with 400 milligrams of SAM-e daily significantly reduced depressive symptoms in half of them within a week—and without any severe side effects.

Even though SAM-e works fast, if you are depressed, you must continue to take it, lest you suffer a relapse. Dr. Brown advises taking it for at least six to nine months.

Few Side Effects

A huge drawback of prescription antidepressants is their miserable side effects, including sexual dysfunction, weight gain, dry mouth, blurred vision, constipation, bladder problems, dizziness, headache, drowsiness, nausea, insomnia, and agitation. Obviously, this makes people not want to take them. In fact, 30 percent of people in clinical trials stop taking them, making the actual success rate of prescription antidepressants only 40 percent.

In contrast, SAM-e has none of these side effects, says Dr. Brown, and is nontoxic, even in high doses. Indeed, in studies SAM-e produced no more side effects than a placebo or sugar pill. Is there any downside to SAM-e? Yes, says Dr. Brown. SAM-e could exacerbate the manic phase of manic depression (bipolar disorder); thus, people with bipolar disorder should take SAM-e only under the close supervision of a psychiatrist, advises Dr. Brown. SAM-e has no known harmful interactions with other medications, including prescription antidepressants and St. John's wort. However, don't combine MAO inhibitor-type antidepressants and SAM-e, just in case, cautions Dr. Brown, and inform your doctor about what you are taking.

How Much?

A typical effective dose for most people with mild to moderate depression is 400 milligrams a day, according to Drs. Brown and Bottiglieri. If you don't see a 25 percent improvement within two weeks, they suggest upping the dose of SAM-e to 800 milligrams a day. If you have a history of sensitivity to medications, start with 200 milligrams for the first week. They also suggest taking SAM-e on an empty stomach a half-hour before meals; if you experience heartburn, take it with meals.

Where to get it? SAM-e is available in bottles or blister

packs from health food stores, drugstores, and discount stores. Be sure to look for "enteric coated," meaning it is best absorbed and most stable.

BOTTOM LINE: *SAM-e appears to be a good alternative to prescription drugs for treating mild depression. At about seventy-five dollars per month, it is less expensive than prescription drugs, but more expensive than St. John's wort.*

Caution: It can be dangerous to self-diagnose depression and take supplements on your own without a doctor's advice. Do not take such supplements along with antidepressant drugs without consulting a physician. If you are more than mildly depressed (stressed out, down in the dumps, under the weather with fatigue, mild anxiety, lack of zest, less fun in life, less productive and creative than usual), see a health professional for an accurate diagnosis. More serious depression may be related to physical causes (brain tumor or malfunctioning thyroid) and may require additional medical treatment.

PART 4

HOW TO KEEP VASCULAR VILLAINS FROM DESTROYING YOUR BRAIN

If it affects your heart, it affects your brain. These two organs are inextricably linked by miles of arteries, blood vessels, and capillaries that feed your heart and also go up into your skull to feed your brain. Thus, damage to the blood-oxygen-glucose transportation system reverberates not only in the heart but also in the brain. The same thing that clogs large arteries and can stop hearts also tends to clog and damage brain blood conduits, including tiny brain capillaries, inflicting disability and death on brain cells.

The molecular stuff transported through your blood vessels, such as cholesterol, triglycerides, and toxic homocysteine—can affect intelligence, memory, mood, vulnerability to stroke and intellectual decline. Research even shows that mini-strokes, and inflammation of cerebral vessels are implicated in Alzheimer's disease, accentuating intellectual losses. Thus, so-called "vascular dementia" (mainly thought due to tiny strokes) and Alzheimer's-type dementia are not isolated, as once thought, but intertwined. In fact, severe cardiovascular disease increases your risk of Alzheimer's.

Indeed, if you can stay free of serious heart disease, you dramatically slash your risk of memory loss and dementia as you get older. Additionally, avoiding diabetes and Alzheimer's practically guarantees you a normally functioning brain in old age.

> **BOTTOM LINE:** *Only recently have scientists begun to understand how vascular villains conspire to harm your brain, and how critical it is to protect your brain from the ravages of cardiovascular disease. Taking extra measures to prevent heart disease and diabetes may have an enormous payoff—a well-functioning, nondemented brain until the end of life.*

BAD ARTERIES, BAD BRAIN

Over the last few years research has increasingly tied blood vessel abnormalities—high blood pressure, high blood sugar, thickened carotid arteries—to intellectual decline as you get older. Now a new landmark study defines precisely how crucial such factors are in keeping your mind intact. For ten years, Mary N. Haan and colleagues at the University of California at Davis School of Medicine tracked 5,888 persons over age sixty-five, testing their mental capabilities every year. The troubling finding: Severe atherosclerosis tripled the risk of decline in mental function—including all aspects of cognition—perception, thinking, reasoning, memory, speed of mental processing—as measured by standard tests. Most profoundly detrimental were high systolic blood pressure, atrial fibrillation (irregular heartbeat), greater thickness of the wall of carotid (neck) arteries, congestive heart failure, and strokes. Those with diabetes and glucose intolerance also showed signs of accelerated mental decline.

Another factor strongly determined cognitive decline: About 25 percent of the study group carried a gene (so-called apolipoprotein E4 gene) associated with Alzheimer's disease. This gene tripled or quadrupled the risk of loss of mental function. Worst of all was a combination of severe cardiovascular disease or diabetes and the gene. People with that combination were eight times more apt to suffer mental decline as those with little atherosclerosis or diabetes and no genetic abnormality.

This means that cardiovascular disease or diabetes alone can dramatically increase your odds of mind slippage with age. The good news is it also suggests that a genetic predisposition to Alzheimer's may not kick in unless you also have cardiovascular disease or diabetes. However, the magnitude of the threat is alarming. It indicates that serious heart disease and diabetes may be a prelude to or stimulant of severe, irreversible intellectual erosion in one-quarter of all adults who unknowingly carry the gene. If you did not already have incentive enough to try to ward off heart disease, this may be a reason that convinces you. Where the heart goes, the brain follows.

Here's the latest scientific evidence on specific blood factors that can damage your brain.

Beware Homocysteine—Potent Brain Toxin

An amino acid in your blood that few doctors even knew about until very recently is now considered a major factor in brain breakdown. It's called homocysteine, and too much of it can accumulate in blood, helping clog and destroy blood vessels, including those that feed the brain; it may even damage mental acuity and mood by a direct toxic effect on brain cells. Luckily, homocysteine is a dragon easily slain by modest doses of B vitamins, which makes its continuing human destruction all the more appalling. High homocysteine, like high cholesterol, can be determined by a blood test.

Unquestionably, high homocysteine is incriminated in failing intellectual abilities. Tufts University researchers recently reported that middle-aged to elderly men with the highest homocysteine blood concentrations performed on one test of mental competence exactly like patients with mild Alzheimer's disease! In fact, among the 25 percent with the highest homocysteine, only 22 percent could correctly copy a cube and only 17 percent could copy a tapered box. About 75 percent of those with the lowest homocysteine levels drew the figures correctly, as can most children by age thirteen. Such subnormal performances in older people indicate the brain has been damaged, said researchers.

BRAIN ALERT: As much as 40 percent of cerebrovascular disease appears tied to high homocysteine levels.

High levels of homocysteine signify not only problems with memory, concentration, and thinking abilities, but also to low moods. Among a group of depressed persons, young and old, the higher the homocysteine, the lower the scores on mental acuity and mood assessment tests. In a recent study of outpatients with major depression, 20 percent had elevated homocysteine and 19 percent, low folic acid.

BOTTOM LINE: *High blood levels of homocysteine predict increased susceptibility to mental impairment and depression in both the old and young.*

THE STROKE CONNECTION

Overwhelming evidence shows that high blood homocysteine predicts strokes. A 1992 review of medical research (a meta-analysis) by Swedish researchers found that fully one-quarter of patients with cerebrovascular disease had high homocysteine. Angiograms of the carotid (neck) artery that feeds blood and oxygen to the brain revealed a blockage or closing in fully 85 percent of a group of patients with high homocysteine who had suffered a TIA (a prelude to stroke) or a minor stroke. In fact, homocysteine is a stronger predictor of stroke than *smoking, high blood pressure, or high cholesterol*, revealed a large scale study of stroke victims by Swedish neurologist Dr. Lars E. Brattstrom at University Hospital in Lund. Forty percent who had strokes of all types—from an embolism, hemorrhage, blockage, or carotid artery disease—had high homocysteine.

Similarly, British researchers studying 7,735 middle-aged men over a thirteen-year period found that the higher the homocysteine, the higher the stroke risk—regardless of weight, diabetes, cholesterol, high blood pressure, or smoking! Indeed, those with the highest homocysteine were about three times more apt to have a stroke than those with the lowest levels.

HOMOCYSTEINE PREDICTS ALZHEIMER'S

Also disturbing, high homocysteine is a sign you may be on the fast track for Alzheimer's. A new study by Robert Clarke, M.D., of Oxford University in England, found that a high homocysteine reading raised odds of developing Alzheimer's by an astounding 450 percent! Not surprisingly, those with Alzheimer's also had low blood levels of folic acid and vitamin B_{12}, which suppresses homocysteine. Low levels of folic acid tripled the odds of Alzheimer's.

Even more alarming, the higher the blood homocysteine, the faster Alzheimer's moved to destroy the brain. Homocysteine's power to speed brain deterioration was seen on brain scans and on declining scores on mental and memory tests. Researchers visually charted the wasting away of specific temporal lobes of the Alzheimer's-diseased brains, and the higher the homocysteine, the greater the shrinkage. In those with the highest homocysteine, a specific brain lobe shrank about 20 percent in three years compared with only 5 percent in those with the lowest homocysteine. As expected, the progression of Alzheimer's also was greatest in those with the lowest folic acid and B_{12}.

How homocysteine promotes Alzheimer's disease is not clearly understood, although recent evidence suggests the combination of disease in cerebral blood vessels and Alzheimer's interacts to worsen the brain damage. Further, high homocysteine may be a marker for low folic acid, thought to help protect the brain from Alzheimer's.

> **BRAIN ALERT:** High homocysteine triples your risk of stroke and quadruples your chances of Alzheimer's disease.

How to Zap Homocysteine

The cure for brain-damaging homocysteine is amazingly simple and inexpensive: B vitamins, notably folic acid. The absence of folic acid allows toxic homocysteine to pile up wildly in the blood. Folic acid breaks it down. Vitamins B_6 and B_{12} also help dispose of homocysteine, but folic acid is by far the most powerful suppresser. Harvard investigators determined that at least two-thirds of high homocysteine is linked to low levels of folic acid. People who take multivitamins, typically containing 400 micrograms of folic acid, have much lower homocysteine than nonvitamin users.

Taking B vitamins can even stop and reverse homocysteine's purported damage to vital carotid arteries, according to a groundbreaking 1998 study by Canadian cardiologist J. David Spence, M.D., at the University of Toronto. He and colleagues measured the progressive closure and plaque buildup in the carotid neck arteries of thirty-eight men and women, average age fifty-eight, before and after taking B vitamins for four and a half years. The results were astonishing.

When not taking B vitamins, the subjects' plaque area increased about 50 percent. After taking vitamins, the plaque actually decreased in size about 10 percent. In short, the vitamins acted as a kind of detergent to clean out arteries and reverse atherosclerosis. Dr. Spence's study used a high dose of folic acid—2.5 milligrams—because a few people need that much to overcome a genetic predisposition to extra high homocysteine. However, he says 400 micrograms of folic acid—a typical daily dose—curbs high homocysteine in most people. He also gave 250 micrograms B_{12} and 25 milligrams of B_6.

Why is high homocysteine a villain in blood vessel and brain tissue damage? One theory: Homocysteine sets the stage in blood vessel linings for clotting and deposition of plaque, leading to damage and closure of vessels. In particular, homocysteine incites artery cells to synthesize collagen, a major component in atherosclerotic plaques, which may also cause stiffening of the blood vessel. Second, homocysteine may block the synthesis of neurotransmitters, such as serotonin. Third, high homocysteine may act as a neurotoxin by triggering metabolic changes resulting in activation of substances, such as glutamate, that directly injure and kill brain cells.

BRAIN ALERT: Only one in ten Americans gets the amount of folic acid needed to curb high homocysteine, according to Harvard researchers.

EGGS AND HOMOCYSTEINE

Ironically, public health warnings against eggs, because of their high cholesterol, may actually aggravate the homocysteine problem. Egg yolks are one of the best sources of choline, a B vitamin. Studies in the 1950s showed that depriving animals of choline caused homocysteine levels to soar. Thus, shunning eggs in attempts to avoid heart disease may in fact have worsened the risk by promoting high homocysteine levels. As it turns out, dietary cholesterol, as in eggs, is not a primary culprit in raising blood cholesterol. (For more on how choline protects the brain, see page 284.)

High Triglycerides Disturb Mood

You may know that high triglycerides, a type of fat in your blood, can be hazardous to your heart. But it's not widely known that high triglycerides can also be detrimental to your brain, says Dr. Charles Glueck, medical director of the Cholesterol Center of Jewish Hospital in Cincinnati. His compelling research has found that high triglycerides are closely tied to depression, hostility, aggression, and even hyperactivity in children. In fact, Dr. Glueck says high triglycerides cause oxygen deficiencies in the brain that can lead to mini-lesions and blood clots that look for all the world like so-called "organic brain syndrome."

In a 1993 study, Dr. Glueck showed that lowering triglycerides can dramatically boost mood and combat depression. Among a group of twenty-three men and women with high triglycerides, about 40 percent were

FIVE WAYS TO LOWER BRAIN-BUSTING HOMOCYSTEINE

- Take folic acid, B_6, and B_{12} supplements. Experts generally advise 400 micrograms of folic acid a day to squelch homocysteine. Dutch investigators recently found that 250 micrograms of folic acid lowered homocysteine by 11 percent in younger women, and 500 micrograms reduced it by 22 percent. It worked best against the highest levels of homocysteine. Another large study found that people taking multiple vitamins with 400 micrograms of folic acid had 10 to 15 percent lower homocysteine than non-vitamin-takers. A few people with genetic factors may need higher doses, prescribed by a doctor. Most experts say 25 milligrams of B_6 and 250 micrograms of B_{12} are generally enough to suppress homocysteine.

  To keep a lid on homocysteine, you must continue to take B vitamins. Stopping causes homocysteine to shoot up to abnormal levels again within four months or so.

- Eat foods high in folic acid, such as orange juice, legumes, green leafy vegetables, almonds, fortified cereals, and avocados. However, your body utilizes only half as much folic acid from food as from supplements. A recent study found that eating high folic acid foods alone did not adequately suppress high homocysteine in about two-thirds of a group of elderly subjects. Thus, folic acid supplements are essential.

- Restrict coffee to less than five cups daily. Recent Norwegian research found that homocysteine was 20 percent higher in people who drank more than nine cups of coffee compared with less than one cup daily. More than five cups daily may raise homocysteine, research suggests. Those who both smoked and drank lots of coffee had particularly high homocysteine.
- Go easy on meat. The body makes homocysteine from high protein foods, notably animal protein, explains Kilmer S. McCully, M.D., at the Veterans Affairs Medical Center in Providence and originator of the homocysteine theory. Protein-rich plant foods are okay because they usually contain enough B vitamins to curb homocysteine, he adds.
- *Don't smoke. Smoking suppresses folic acid levels, paving the way for excessive formation of homocysteine.

mildly to severely depressed, according to standard criteria. After a year on a triglyceride-lowering diet and drugs, their average triglycerides dropped nearly 50 percent, and their depression virtually disappeared. Fully 91 percent of the formerly depressed returned to normal, most within six weeks, says Dr. Glueck. More impressive, the greater the fall in triglycerides, the greater the improvement in mood.

Dr. Glueck also studied 220 children ages five to eighteen who were hospitalized with mood disorders, schizophrenia, anxiety, and organic psychiatric disorders. Those with disruptive behavior and attention deficit hyperactivity disorder had higher triglycerides than a group of normal children.

A string of other evidence incriminates triglycerides in brain disturbances and behavior. British researchers found that men with abnormally high triglycerides tend to have denigratory attitudes toward women, are more apt to commit hostile acts and have a "domineering" attitude. Brandeis University psychologists have linked high triglycerides to "cognitive impairment," including depression and memory problems among some diabetics. As triglycerides rose over a five-year-period, so did hostility in a group of young men ages twenty-three to thirty-five, reported University of Alabama investigators in 1997.

Unquestionably, high triglycerides are now viewed as a major villain in blood-clot (ischemic) strokes, according to several studies. Japanese researchers noted that middle-aged diabetics with high triglycerides were twice as likely to suffer a stroke.

How do high triglycerides undermine the brain? Dr. Glueck says excessive triglycerides make blood sluggish, more apt to form small clots, cutting down blood and oxygen to brain cells. Dr. Robert Rosenson, at Rush Medical College in Chicago, has found that triglycerides at levels above 190 milligrams per deciliter make blood strikingly more viscous and clot-prone. High triglycerides also are tied to the most menacing type of cholesterol, small, dense LDL particles, most apt to infiltrate blood vessel walls and promote clogging. High triglycerides also are an integral part of an "insulin resistance syndrome," which destroys arteries, foreshadows diabetes, and is detrimental to mental function. Although 200 milligrams per deciliter has been considered a relatively safe triglyceride level, many experts now consider 100 or less an "ideal" level.

IS IT REALLY THE FISH?

If high triglycerides promote depression, and fish oil lowers triglycerides, could that be one way fish oil fights depression? "Yes, I think that's a logical connection," says NIH depression and fish oil expert Dr. Joseph Hibbeln.

HOW TO REDUCE BRAIN-DAMAGING TRIGLYCERIDES

Eat seafood and/or take fish oil supplements. Omega–3 fish oil is the most effective, safest way to lower triglycerides—better than any known drug—according to experts. After reviewing seventy-two studies, William Harris, Ph.D., director of the Lipoprotein Research Laboratory, St. Luke's Hospital in Kansas City, concluded that a daily 3,000 to 4,000 milligrams of fish oil cut high triglycerides an average 28 percent. Another study found a daily dose—comparable to eating seven ounces of salmon, mackerel, or sardines—slashed triglycerides more than 50 percent. And it works quickly—usually normalizing triglyceride levels within a couple of weeks.

Even substituting shellfish for the usual meat, eggs, milk, and cheese protein, may send triglycerides down dramatically, according to a University of Washington study. Triglycerides sank 61 percent in clam-eaters, 51 percent in oyster-eaters, and 23 percent in crab-eaters.

Restrict alcohol. It can raise triglycerides. One or two drinks a day are usually not a problem.

Curb your intake of carbohydrates, especially refined sugar, including fructose-sweetened soft drinks. Studies show that sugar raises triglycerides far more than starchy complex carbohydrates such as bread, potatoes, and pasta.

In people who are "insulin resistant" (usually indicated by high triglycerides and low good-type HDL cholesterol), sugar-rich diets send triglycerides skyrocketing. To keep triglycerides in check, whole fruit is better than fruit juices; whole grain, high-fiber starches are better than low-fiber "convenience foods" such as chips, and low-fat, high-sugar "diet" cookies and candies.

High Blood Pressure Harms Memory

A major threat to your brain as you get older is a stroke, often triggered by high blood pressure. Moreover, high blood pressure, even in the absence of a stroke, often inflicts subtle brain damage that can erode mental faculties.

High blood pressure today, memory loss tomorrow, is the message from recent research that links high blood pressure to damaged brain tissue, cognitive impairment, and "vascular dementia"—a decline in mental functioning, including memory, usually from vessel damage or ministrokes.

In a 1998 study of 999 men, Swedish researchers at the Karolinska Hospital in Stockholm clearly documented that high blood pressure "can lead to cognitive impairment." Men, now in their fifties, who had high blood pressure readings twenty years ago, showed the greatest decline in mental capacity and motor skills when recently tested. Men with the highest diastolic (lower number) blood pressure reading—over 105 mm/Hg—had the greatest mental impairment. Men with the lowest diastolic pressure—less than 70 mm/Hg—scored highest in thinking ability. Men whose high blood pressure had gone untreated suffered the most decline.

This study jibes with findings from an ongoing collaborative research at Stanford, UCLA, Indiana University, and

Boston University. Researchers have tied high systolic (upper number) blood pressure in middle age to sharper declines in mental acuity after age sixty. For example men who had systolic pressure above 140 for twenty-five years exhibited twice as much intellectual decline as men with normal blood pressure. The suspected reason: The men had probably already experienced small undetected (silent) strokes induced by their high blood pressure.

HIGH BLOOD PRESSURE SHRINKS BRAINS

Indeed, high blood pressure can accelerate brain shrinkage as you age. This may help explain intellectual decline typical of old-age brain deterioration not caused by Alzheimer's, according to researchers at the National Institute on Aging. They used brain imaging scans and neuropsychological tests to study people ages fifty-six to eighty-four, some with high blood pressure, others with normal blood pressure.

Investigators detected startling brain differences, even though none of the high blood pressure patients had ever had a stroke. The scans revealed that high blood pressure had taken a toll in increased brain atrophy in the temporal and occipital lobes that control memory and language. Those with high blood pressure also scored lower on language and memory tests than same-age individuals with normal blood pressure. "And the effect worsened with age," said senior investigator Gene E. Alexander. The older the person, the worse the loss of brain matter and function. Unfortunately, taking drugs to control high blood pressure did not totally prevent detrimental brain changes.

More recently, Charles DeCarli, M.D., associate professor of neurology and director of the Alzheimer's Disease Center at the University of Kansas, used magnetic resonance imaging (MRI) to document that midlife high blood pressure speeds up aging and shrinkage of the brain, increasing risk of stroke in late life.

He tracked 414 individuals, starting when they were average age forty-seven for about twenty-five years. Specifically, he found that those with high blood pressure in midlife had smaller brains, more abnormal white matter (specific nerve tissue in the brain), and a higher risk of stroke, including silent strokes, in old age. Such "silent strokes" occur in the tiny blood vessels of the brain without symptomatic fanfare, but over time result in subtle progressive damage, usually detectable only by an MRI. (About 12 percent in his study showed signs of silent strokes on brain imaging.) Further, "the higher your blood pressure, in midlife, the worse the outlook for old age—the smaller your brain, the more extensive the white matter damage and the greater the expected intellectual impairment," says Dr. DeCarli.

Distressingly, even borderline high blood pressure at midlife predicted greater brain atrophy in old age. Dr. DeCarli worries that many middle-aged people who appear healthy may, in fact, have borderline high blood pressure that is slowly, but surely, sabotaging their brains. So potentially devastating is the damage that he urges everyone with even borderline high blood pressure to find ways to reduce it.

"People with high blood pressure are four times more apt to have a stroke." —Dr. Philip Wolf, professor of neurology, Boston University

Even slight blood pressure elevations may help precipitate a stroke. Indeed, Boston University investigators recently found in a study of 566 people over a forty-year period that half of the strokes occurred in those with high normal (defined as 130–139 mmHg systolic, the top number) or mildly high blood pressure (140–159 mmHg systolic).

What about caffeine? Dr. Jack E. James, LaTrobe University, Melbourne, Australia, says that coffee increases blood pressure in the population on average by 2 to 4 mm Hg. Thus, cutting out caffeine, he predicts, could reduce stroke risk by 17 to 24 percent.

ALCOHOL: A BLOOD PRESSURE HAZARD

Many experts call alcohol a widespread but largely unrecognized cause of high blood pressure. Some studies show that excessive drinking makes blood pressure soar, and that cutting back to moderate consumption may help. But new research suggests that drinking no alcohol at all is the best way to lower blood pressure. In one new study directed mostly at African-Americans, researchers found that drinking only one drink of alcohol per day significantly boosted both diastolic and systolic blood pressure.

Government researchers who conducted the famous blood-pressure-reducing DASH Diet also concluded that abstaining from alcohol is more apt to lower your blood pressure than drinking moderately.

PREVENT STROKE, PREVENT ALZHEIMER'S

Although most people fear Alzheimer's disease far more than stroke, in reality you should find the possibility of stroke more terrifying. A stroke is much more likely to strike and be more destructive and, in fact, tiny strokes may be the precipitating factor that pushes your brain over the brink into severe brain failure or Alzheimer's. In a groundbreaking study, published in the *Journal of the American Medical Association* in March, 1997, Dr. David Snowdon, noted brain researcher at the University of Kentucky, reported the astonishing news that one or two small strokes

SIX NON-DRUG WAYS TO REDUCE BLOOD PRESSURE

- Take 1000 milligrams vitamin C daily. U.S. Department of Agriculture research showed that six weeks of vitamin C supplementation shaved an average 8 to 10 points off systolic readings and an average 7 points off diastolic readings in those with borderline high blood pressure. It even decreased normal blood pressure.

- Cut sodium intake to no more than 2400 milligrams a day. Best way, cut down on highly salted processed foods with hidden sodium. Check the label.

- If overweight, take off pounds. A slight loss of only ten pounds can have an impact. Excessive weight is the most prevalent cause of high blood pressure. A recent analysis of many studies found that weight loss was almost twice as effective as other dietary measures in reducing blood pressure. Losing weight depressed systolic blood pressure by 5.2 points compared with 2.9 points for salt restriction.

- Avoid alcohol entirely is the most effective advice. Otherwise, at least limit yourself to two drinks a day if you're a man or one drink per day if a woman.

- Get regular physical exercise—such as half an hour to an hour of brisk walking every day.

- Eat fruits and vegetables. It's clear, say Harvard nutritionists, that chemicals and fiber in fruits and vegetables lower blood pressure. One Israeli study of two hundred people showed that only 2 percent of vegetarians had high blood pressure compared with 26 percent of meat eaters.

in strategic parts of the brain boosts your chances of Alzheimer's-type dementia twenty times over! His insights, gained from studying the structure and functioning of the brains of a large group of elderly nuns after death (the so-called Nun's Study), suggest that Alzheimer's-type plaques and strokes damage different specific regions of the brain, and that together they produce a synergistic whammy—worse damage and dementia than either alone. "Stroke plus Alzheimer's is not one plus one equals two. It's more like one plus one equals four or five," says Dr. Snowdon.

Amazingly, your brain can show evidence of Alzheimer's damage, but if a stroke does not come along, your brain may continue to function fairly normally—with little intellectual decline, memory loss, or so-called dementia. Such "tiny strokes may be the switch that flips a mildly deteriorating brain into full-fledged dementia" as *Time* magazine put it. In short: "If you remain stroke-free, you can handle more lesions of Alzheimer's," says Dr. Snowdon. He speculates that a stroke on top of Alzheimer's injuries simply potentiates brain cell destruction. Widespread inflammation was also present in the brains of those most severely affected intellectually.

Dr. Snowdon's discovery is important because there are strategies to prevent strokes, whereas there are only promising, but uncertain ways to stop the initial brain injuries of Alzheimer's. The idea, then, says Dr. Snowdon, is to stop the progression of Alzheimer's damage by preventing strokes. Even postponing Alzheimer's dementia by five years would slash in half the number of people with overt symptoms of the disease, he says.

BOTTOM LINE: *Reduce your odds of stroke and you stay many steps away from Alzheimer's and the consequent intellectual downslide known as dementia.*

ASTONISHING WAY TO AVOID AND SURVIVE A STROKE

One antistroke secret is simple: Eat fruits and vegetables, drink tea. It's strikingly clear that eating fruits and vegetables helps prevent strokes and lessen damage should you suffer a stroke. Medical researchers have been screaming this message for more than two decades. It's a mystery why fruits and vegetables are such powerful stroke-fighters; it could be their high antioxidants, potassium, folic acid, or many factors combined. But the evidence is so utterly compelling that the first thing you should do to avoid stroke is eat more fruits and vegetables.

As part of the large-scale Framingham Study, Harvard researchers followed 832 men, ages forty-five to sixty-five for twenty years; the more fruit and vegetables the men ate, the less likely they were to have a stroke or a warning sign of stroke, a TIA (transient ischemic attack). In fact, increasing intake of fruits and vegetables by three servings per day reduced overall stroke rates 22 percent and risk of hemorraghic or bleeding stroke by 51 percent! A serving is one fruit or vegetable or one-half cup. The fruits and vegetables had an impact unrelated to blood pressure, cholesterol, smoking, drinking, exercise, or fat or calorie intake. In short, some magical ingredients in fruits and vegetables appear to help protect against stroke regardless of what else you do. In this study, vegetables had more antistroke power than fruits.

Women, too, slash stroke risk by eating fruits and vegetables, particularly carrots, according to a previous Harvard study that tracked 90,000 women nurses for eight years. Just eating slightly less than a carrot a day cut the odds of stroke in the women an astounding 68 percent compared with eating carrots only once a month! Eating spinach also dramatically deterred strokes. A common stroke-fighting element in the vegetables could be the antioxidant beta-carotene, said researcher JoAnn E. Manson, M.D., of Brigham and Women's Hospital and Harvard Medical School.

A more recent thirty-year look at 1,843 men (middle-aged when the study started) found that those who ate fruits and vegetables with the most beta-carotene and vitamin C were least apt to have nonfatal or fatal stroke. Indeed, the highest intake of beta-carotene decreased risk about 15 percent compared with the lowest intake. And vitamin C suppressed stroke risk about 30 percent.

Another brain-protecting miracle agent in fruits and vegetables and tea are flavonoids—non-nutrient chemicals, such as quercetin and catechins and pigments. Dutch researchers found that those who ate the most flavonoids in fruits, vegetables, and tea were 73 percent less likely to suffer a stroke than those eating the least flavonoids. In this case, black tea was the biggest contributor to antistroke flavonoids in the diet. Drinking about five cups of tea a day versus two-and-a-half cups per day reduced the risk of stroke 70 percent.

THE AMAZING POTASSIUM PROTECTION

Another secret ingredient of fruits and vegetables is potassium, and eating a little extra potassium (also in fish and milk) may save you from a deadly stroke. The evidence is consistent and compelling. A pioneering classic study a decade ago in California came to the stunning conclusion that just an extra serving of a potassium-rich food (400 milligrams) every day reduced the risk of fatal stroke by a startling 40 percent! A mere extra banana or apple or half cup of spinach a day spelled the difference between life and death. By analyzing the diets of 859 men and women over age fifty, Dr. Kay Tee Khaw, and colleagues at the University of California, documented that the intake of potassium predicted who was most apt to have a stroke twelve years later.

Among those who ate the least potassium (less than 1950 milligrams per day) compared with those who ate the most (more than 3500 milligrams a day), the risk of fatal stroke skyrocketed 2.6 times in men and 4.8 times in women. The protective difference: only 400 milligrams of potassium a day. Further, the more potassium foods the subjects ate, the more their stroke risk dropped.

And there's more evidence that potassium may save you from stroke:

Harvard researchers tracked 43,738 male health professionals for eight years and recently noted that those who took in the most potassium in foods and supplements had the lowest rates of stroke. Men in the top 20 percent of potassium intake were 38 percent less apt to have a stroke than those in the lowest 20 percent. Lowest-risk men ate about eight servings of fruits and vegetables a day, twice that of men with the highest stroke risk. Moreover, men who took diuretics for high blood pressure and also took potassium supplements (about 1000 milligrams daily) were 64 percent less apt to have a stroke than diuretic takers who did not take potassium.

One of the most persuasive recent studies measured blood levels of potassium in 824 men and women participating in the Northern Manhattan Stroke Study. Those with the highest blood potassium were 40 percent less likely to have a stroke.

Researchers at the University of Minnesota find that potassium does more to fight strokes than just lower blood pressure. Potassium also protects the lining of blood vessels, the endothelium, against free-radical damage in animals with high blood pressure. Thus, potassium may directly combat high-blood-pressure-induced damage to arteries, making them less susceptible to a stroke.

WHAT TO EAT TO ESCAPE STROKES

Each of these foods provides the extra 400 milligrams of daily potassium shown to slash the odds of fatal stroke by 40 percent.

- 1/2 cup cooked fresh spinach (423 milligrams)
- 1/2 cup cooked fresh beet greens (654 milligrams)
- 1 tsp. blackstrap molasses (400 milligrams)
- 1 cup tomato juice (536 milligrams)
- 1 cup fresh orange juice (472 milligrams)
- 1/4 cantaloupe (412 milligrams)
- 1/2 cup acorn squash (446 milligrams)
- 10 dried apricot halves (482 milligrams)
- 2 carrots (466 milligrams)
- 1/2 cup cooked sweet potato (455 milligrams)
- 1/2 cup cooked green lima beans (484 milligrams)
- 1 cup skim milk (418 milligrams)
- 1/2 Florida avocado (742 milligrams)
- 1 banana (451 milligrams)
- 2 ounces almonds (440 milligrams)
- 1 ounce roasted soybeans (417 milligrams)
- 17-ounce baked potato without skin (512 milligrams)
- 17-ounce baked potato with skin (844 milligrams)
- 1/2 cup baked beans (613 milligrams)
- 3 ounces (about eight) canned sardines (500 milligrams)
- 3 ounces swordfish steak (465 milligrams)

Reprinted from *Food—Your Miracle Medicine*

ALCOHOL: THE HARM AND BENEFIT

Decidedly, drinking too much alcohol for too long can bring on a stroke. Drinking seven or more drinks a day triples your risk of having an ischemic (blood clot) stroke, according to new research by Ralph L. Sacco, Columbia University College of Physicians and Surgeons in New York, who studied 677 stroke victims aged forty and older. However, he says heavy drinkers can reverse their higher risk by reducing intake to two drinks a day or quitting drinking entirely. On the other hand, moderate drinkers—up to two drinks per day—had a 45 percent lower risk of blood-clot stroke when compared with nondrinkers.

Other studies show that heavy drinking dramatically raises the risk of a bleeding or hemorrhagic stroke. Further, the amount of alcohol you drink may help determine the size of a stroke. The more you drink, the larger and more damaging the stroke, according to one recent analysis. Binge drinking is particularly risky, sometimes triggering strokes, even in young people.

WINE VS. STROKES

There's new evidence that people who drink wine appear to have a lower risk of strokes. Danish researcher Thomas Truelsen, M.D., at Copenhagen University Hospital, in a large study of thirteen thousand men and women over a period of sixteen years, found stroke odds 34 percent lower in those who drank one to six glasses of wine a week compared with those who drank wine not at all or infrequently. (About two-thirds of the wine consumed in Denmark is red wine.) Moderate drinkers of spirits had a 3 percent lower stroke risk. People who drank beer once a week or more had a 9 percent greater chance of suffering a stroke. As expected, heavy drinking was harmful. Six drinks a day or more raised stroke risk 50 percent.

How Much?

Moderate drinking is defined as one or two drinks per day for men and one drink for women and those older than age sixty-five. One drink is: a 12-ounce bottle of beer or a wine cooler; a 5-ounce glass of wine, or 1.5 ounces 80-proof distilled spirits.

> *"The issue of alcohol intake and disease prevention is a tricky one for physicians, who do not recommend that anyone take up drinking for his or her health. The physical and emotional damage wrought by alcohol abuse in this country is enormous, and light or moderate drinking is not possible for many people. . . . But because . . . alcohol appears to play a role in preventing [heart disease] and now stroke, physicians advise people who drink small amounts to keep doing what they are doing . . . everything in moderation."*
> —*Harvard Health Letter*, March 1999

Drinking seven or more drinks a day triples your risk of having an ischemic (blood clot) stroke. Former heavy drinkers who restrict drinking to no more than two drinks per day or quit entirely erase the added risk of stroke.

BOTTOM LINE: *Drinking in moderation (one drink a day for women, no more than two for men), especially red wine, might help discourage a blood-clot type stroke. Heavy drinking or binge drinking is sure to be detrimental, helping bring on a stroke, especially a bleeding stroke. However, if you do not currently drink alcohol, do not start drinking as an anti-stroke measure. Considering the downside of alcohol, there are* *many other safer ways to care for your brain and body, that can have a much greater impact in deterring a stroke.*

SALT, STROKE, AND BLOOD PRESSURE

Overdosing on salt or sodium can boost blood pressure and stroke risk in many, but not all, people. Some, for genetic reasons, are more "salt sensitive," meaning their vascular system reacts more vigorously when loaded with salt. If you are overweight, the odds are worse. Tulane University researchers recently found that an increase in sodium of a mere 100 mmol a day doubled the risk of fatal strokes among 2700 overweight men and women.

Japan is a striking case in point. Historically, the Japanese consume extraordinary amounts of sodium, for example in soy sauce and salted fish. They also historically have one of the highest rates of stroke in the world, particularly hemorrhagic or bleeding strokes. High sodium makes blood vessels in the brain more permeable and leaky, say

---

DON'T DRINK ALCOHOL IF YOU:

- Are pregnant or considering pregnancy.
- Have a medical condition that can be worsened by drinking such as an ulcer or liver disease
- Have a personal or family history of alcoholism
- Are taking medication that may interact with alcohol
- Are planning to drive or engage in other activities that require you to be alert
- Are under the legal drinking age.

SOURCE: American Medical Association

---

experts, and vulnerable to ruptures, spilling blood into the brain. A recent nationwide health initiative to lower blood pressure and intake of sodium has led to a decided drop in strokes among the Japanese, for the first time in recent history.

Cholesterol: Good and Bad

There's plenty of evidence that blood cholesterol is heavily involved in atherosclerosis that clogs and stiffens the blood conduits of the body, the cerebral blood vessels as well as coronary arteries. The worst appears to be LDL (low density lipoprotein) cholesterol that when "oxidized" (turned rancid by free-radical chemicals) is able to infiltrate blood vessel walls and accelerate plaque buildup, eventually reducing blood flow and encouraging release of blood clots.

It's known, for example, that high levels of bad-type LDL blood cholesterol are tied to greater susceptibility to strokes as well as heart attacks. A recent study by Canadian neurologists at London Health Sciences Centre–University Campus in Ontario, documented that stroke risk goes up along with rises in total cholesterol and bad-type LDL cholesterol in particular. High triglycerides also pushed up stroke chances. On the other hand, investigators found that having high levels of good-type HDL cholesterol reduced the odds of stroke, just as it does heart attacks.

Several studies confirm that high good-type HDL cholesterol may help you evade a stroke, notably the most common "ischemic" or blood-clot caused strokes. Urhan Goldbourt, at the Sheba Medical Center in Tel-Hashomer, Israel, studied 8586 men for twenty-one years. Decidedly, men with the lowest HDL cholesterol—below 35.5 milligrams per deciliter (mg/dl) were 32 percent more likely to have a stroke then men with the highest HDLs—above 42.5 mg/dl. "Blood HDL cholesterol should be considered

WALK AWAY FROM A STROKE

Exciting new evidence shows that moderately intense physical exercise can cut your chances of having a stroke by an astounding 50 percent. That means an hour-long brisk walk five days a week or a comparable expenditure of energy, according to Harvard and Stanford researchers who studied 11,130 Harvard alumni for a dozen years. Compared with men who did little or no exercise, those who expended 2,000 kilocalories a week—equivalent to walking briskly for an hour five days a week—had a 46 percent lower risk of stroke. Walking briskly for half an hour five days a week—or the equivalent—cut the odds of stroke by 24 percent.

Why? Researchers speculate such physical activity reduces blood clotting, lowers cholesterol, reduces blood pressure and weight, all factors related to promoting strokes. Although the study was done on men, researchers say it's logical to think it holds true for women, too.

"Walking, stair-climbing, and participating in moderately intense activities such as dancing, bicycling and gardening were shown to reduce the risk of stroke."—I-Min Lee, M.D., Harvard School of Public Health

a risk factor for stroke," he declared. However, he added that high blood pressure poses a greater stroke threat than low HDLs.

CHOLESTEROL AND ALZHEIMER'S

Bad-type LDL cholesterol is even incriminated in Alzheimer's disease, recent evidence reveals. LDL cholesterol encourages the deposition of a protein called beta amyloid, a major component of senile plaques that characterize Alzheimer's. This beta amyloid is thought to be a major instigator of brain cell deterioration in the disease. This connection between bad cholesterol and beta amyloid might help explain why Alzheimer's brains worsen in the presence of diseased blood vessels.

High cholesterol may be linked to low-level chronic inflammation, now recognized as extremely detrimental to blood vessels and brain tissue. Indeed, Harvard investigators in 1997 found that people with high levels of a blood protein reflecting increased inflammation were twice as apt to have a stroke. The protein is called C-reactive protein (CRP); it's a measurable chemical marker in the blood that goes up as inflammation worsens.

Remarkably, follow-up 1999 research by Harvard cardiologist Paul Ridker, finds that a major way cholesterol-lowering drugs work to fight heart disease is by combating inflammation. During a five year double-blind study patients taking one of the "statin" anticholesterol drugs, pravastatin (Pravachol), had 38 percent lower levels of the CRP inflammatory protein than those who took a placebo pill. The anti-inflammatory benefits were totally independent of the blood cholesterol levels. What causes the inflammation is a mystery, although, says Ridker, "atherosclerosis may ultimately prove to be an inflammatory disease in the same way that we currently consider rheumatoid arthritis to be an inflammatory condition."

BOTTOM LINE: *Keeping your blood vessels healthy is a powerful way to keep your brain healthy.*

Getting the Miracle Brain You Deserve— Ten Top Strategies

Your brain is wonderfully malleable, a treasure to be molded and nurtured throughout life, from birth to old age, as affirmed by the exciting new research reported in this book. There is every reason to believe your brain can give you a lifetime of happiness, intellectual vigor, and satisfying achievements based on the new concept of the brain as a growing, changing organ sculpted by environmental influences, most profoundly by the nutrients, vitamins, and supplements that nourish it every day.

Unfortunately, the typical American diet is not conducive to creating and supporting superior brains. On the other hand, a look at what we eat suggests that we are doing virtually everything to ruin our brains. We eat the wrong type fats guaranteed to cause disruption in the functioning of our brain cells, perhaps ending in neuronal death. We overeat sugar, dumping excessive glucose—over and above that needed to feed and energize brain cells—into the brain where it reacts with free radicals to literally burn brain cells to death. We eat so many calories and get so little exercise that half of all adult Americans are now categorized as obese. Such calorie overloads create more free radical activity in the brain, condemning brain cells to dysfunction and death. We have turned our brains into a wasteland of free radical activity. We shun exercise that energizes the brain. We skimp on fruits and vegetables, full of antioxidants, that might save our brain cells from malfunction and destruction. With our deficient diets, we cheat ourselves of precious nutrients, such as B vitamins and vitamin E, essential for good mental functioning. We induce subtle and serious damage to our brains because of avoidable clogged blood vessels, high blood pressure, insulin resistance, and high homocysteine. We cheat our infants and children of brain-building foods. We fail to stimulate our brains or those of our children with mental activity that prods the growth of brain cells and their interconnections.

The frontier research that makes up this book dictates that it is imperative to consider the severe jeopardy in which we put ourselves and society by ignoring the health of our brains. Of course, not all the scientific information is in, but more than enough is known to point to the right foods and supplements that can make a dramatic difference in preserving the magnificence of our most precious human asset. The evidence, I think, compels all of us to look on our own brain with new respect and optimism, knowing that its power and destiny are truly up to each of us.

Based on the extensive research, here are ten crucial actions you can take now to preserve and enrich your brain's functioning and health:

1. Take multivitamins.

The evidence is utterly compelling that taking modest doses of a variety of vitamins and minerals is excellent brain insurance: They can preserve and improve intellectual functioning and emotional well-being, most likely at all ages. Pregnant women should take multivitamins with their doctors' advice to help guarantee healthy babies. As many as one-half of ordinary schoolchildren might improve IQ scores by taking multivitamins, according to Dr. David Benton, leading British researcher. Many adolescents and adults eat diets lacking basic vitamins and minerals essential for proper brain function, such as folic acid and selenium; a multivitamin can fill in deficiencies. Remember: Suboptimal brain functioning from such deficiencies is usually subtle and unnoticed, often taken for granted; nor are the deficiencies always apparent on blood tests. A combination of vitamins and minerals, found in multivitamin formulas, can help restore optimal intellectual function and lift mood at the same time.

A multivitamin is absolutely essential for older people who tend to need more nutrient help to support an aging brain. Studies show that older people who take a range of vitamins and minerals, especially for a number of years, have better cognitive function and feel better as they age. B vitamins, especially, are critical in preserving aging brains and preventing dementia and depression in old age. Again, subtle deficiencies, easily corrected by a multivitamin, can rob older people of optimal brain functioning and even help bring on brain disease, including dementia.

2. Take antioxidant vitamins.

Usually taking only a multivitamin-mineral pill is not enough. Most do not contain sufficiently high amounts of powerful brain-protecting vitamin E and vitamin C, for example, let alone important alpha lipoic acid and coenzyme Q10. In some studies, people who took only multivitamins showed a decline in cognitive function with age whereas those who took high doses of individual antioxidants, such as vitamin E, did not. In one recent study, not a single elderly person taking individual tablets of vitamin E or vitamin C developed Alzheimer's disease.

Four antioxidant supplements are absolutely essential: vitamin E, vitamin C, alpha lipoic acid, and coenzyme Q10, says antioxidant authority Dr. Lester Packer at the University of California, Berkeley. He also recommends gingko biloba and Pycnogenol™ as powerful brain protectors. (For recommended doses, see individual chapters, pages 242, 249, 259, 266.) It's far smarter to take several antioxidants instead of just one, he says, because they do not work in isolation; their brain-protecting powers are much stronger when they work together.

Should children take antioxidants in addition to a multivitamin? Yes, says Dr. Packer. He recommends half the usual adult dose of antioxidants for children. After all, the earlier the brain gets antioxidants, the less the expected free-radical damage through the years which may be reflected in old age as memory loss, dementia, and even Alzheimer's disease. Antioxidants can also help stave off chronic diseases such as diabetes, clogged arteries, and high blood pressure, which also over time can harm the brain.

3. Eat foods high in antioxidants.

This means fruits and vegetables, loaded with various antioxidants, some probably not yet even identified. Thrilling new animal experiments at Tufts give a glimpse of the power of antioxidant-packed foods on the brain. Feeding animals common high-antioxidant fruits and vegetables, such as blueberries, spinach, and strawberries, has slowed down brain deterioration, revved up mental faculties and even reversed memory and learning losses in old animals. It's mind-boggling to think such fruits and vegetables can rejuvenate the brain!

Virtually all fruits and vegetables contain antioxidants, but for a list of the most potent, see page 152. It's not difficult to take in high doses of antioxidants in modest amounts of fruits and vegetables. Just three prunes, one cup of mixed blueberries and strawberries, plus 1/2 cup of cooked spinach would put you far over the top for the very highest antioxidant daily intake recommended by authorities.

Generally, highest in antioxidants are brightly colored fruits and berries and green leafy vegetables. Snacking on berries, cherries, grapes, apples, prunes, raisins—instead of or even in addition to the usual chips—could make all the difference in intellectual power and emotional well-being.

4. Drink tea.

It's hard to say enough about the fantastic powers of such a common beverage as plain tea in protecting cells, including brain cells, from damage. As Dr. John Weisburger, renowned scientific researcher, now at the American Health Foundation, has said often: "Tea should be the national health beverage." It's one of the easiest, quickest ways to infuse the body and brain with antioxidants. Put one tea bag in a cup of boiling water. Let it brew for five minutes and drink it. In an instant you have taken in about 1200 ORAC units of antioxidants—about one-third to one-fourth the total daily recommended amounts, according to Tufts University researchers.

Iced tea counts, too. You can simply pour the cup of tea over ice. However—and this is important—you do not get any significant amounts of antioxidants in herbal teas, commercial bottled teas, or powdered tea mixes, according to Tufts analyses. The tea must be made from "real" tea leaves, loose or in bags. Further, you can use either plain black tea (yes, the stuff you see on supermarket shelves, such as Lipton's, Twinings, Bigelow) or more exotic Asian green tea. Although green tea has received much hype for its anticancer chemicals, black tea actually has more total antioxidant activity than green tea, Tufts researchers found. So you don't have to go to green tea to get the benefits.

Suggestion: Try substituting at least one cup of tea a day for your regular coffee. Drink iced tea instead of soft drinks. Order iced tea at restaurants, after asking if it is freshly made from real tea.

5. Avoid bad fats.

You can take the perfectly good brain you were born with and screw up its communication circuits by feeding it the wrong type of fat—at any age, from birth, through childhood and adolescence, middle age and old age. Your brain cannot function optimally on a diet of the wrong fats. Few people realize how critical fatty acids are at the molecular level of brain cells in fostering clear and rapid message transmission and energy production that keeps cells alive and vital. Probably the most dangerous to brain cells is saturated animal fat—so pervasive in fast foods, such as hamburgers and shakes.

Unquestionably, animals fed diets high in saturated animal fat are dumber, with impaired memories and learning ability. Animal fat, other research shows, distorts the normal configuration of nerve cell membranes, stifles the growth of synapses (communication junctions), and disturbs the biochemistry of neurotransmitters, the message carriers. Such fat also tends to promote "insulin resistance" later in life, even in youngsters, which leads to abnormal metabolism of insulin and blood sugar, which the brain depends on as its sole source of energy.

Also detrimental to cells: too much polyunsaturated vegetable oil, such as corn oil (so-called omega-6s), that can set up chronic inflammatory responses in brain tissue, thought to eventually lead to subtle brain damage, strokes, and Alzheimer's disease. Eating trans fatty acids, in processed foods such as most margarines, donuts, and fast-food french fries, also can foster blood vessel damage that is detrimental to blood circulation in the brain. (For a list of bad fats, see page 50.)

6. Get omega-3 type fish oil—from eating fish and/or taking supplements.

The fat your brain most needs is so-called omega-3 found in fish oil. It's the evolutionary stuff that formed your brain, and without it, brain cells cannot possibly function at optimal levels. Developing brains—in the womb, infancy and childhood—especially require omega-3 type fish oil to construct the best neuronal architecture and biochemical wiring. Failure to get enough omega-3 in the early developmental periods can result in lower IQs later in life. Nor can adult brains achieve top cognitive potential without adequate supplies of omega–3 fatty acids. Such fat is needed to spur growth of dendrites and synapses, the neuron's mechanisms for processing messages throughout the brain. One fraction of fish oil, called DHA, has been shown to enhance brain power, memory, and learning and may even prevent and possibly treat Alzheimer's disease.

Omega–3 fat also tells your brain to feel good. It is a mood elevator, preventing and even relieving major depression. It can also help prevent brain damage from alcoholism, and may even be a preventive and treatment for some cases of schizophrenia. Kids and adults with attention deficit disorder and dyslexia may suffer from omega–3 deficiencies, which when corrected, lead to better brain functioning.

Eating fatty fish a couple of times a week—or an ounce or two a day—is enough to keep brain cells happy. The alternative: Take fish oil supplements, especially DHA type supplements.

7. Take brain-boosting supplements.

As you age, your brain may need a boost to counteract subtle declines in memory, possibly from a drop in neurotransmitter activity or damage to neurons from disease or routine attacks by free radical chemicals. Some over-the-counter supplements can help rejuvenate brain cell activity. A favorite is ginkgo biloba, taken by many prominent brain researchers to try to ward off age-related memory loss. Another supplement is phosphatidylserine or PS, reputed to stimulate production of the "memory" neurotransmitter acetylcholine, which may decline as you get older. These are worth a try as a way of preventing or overcoming short-term memory problems, which are a part of normal aging, according to brain researchers. They may or may not work, depending on the nature of the problem and biochemical individuality. Their great upside: Unlike potent pharmaceutical drugs which have severe side effects, over-the-counter brain-boosters have no or only minor side effects. Still, if you are under treatment for disease or are taking medications, you should consult your doctor before taking such supplements, especially to rule out potentially hazardous interactions.

8. Watch sugar, including blood sugar.

Eating too much sugar, and certain other carbohydrates, is not a good idea for brains of any age. Sugar overloads can inspire "insulin resistance," throwing blood sugar (glucose) levels out of whack, as well as causing permanent damage to brain cells, leading to malfunction and death. However, since the brain runs on energy derived mostly from carbohydrates, it's essential to have the right amount of blood sugar available to the brain at every instant to promote memory, learning, other cognitive functions. Best carbohydrates for an optimally functioning brain: those that are digested slowly. (For a list, see pages 128–130.)

9. Restrict calories—lose weight.

Being overweight is not good for your brain. It can foster insulin resistance, high blood pressure, and possibly diabetes—leading to impaired memory, accelerated aging, and subtle damage to brain cells. The one sure-fire way to slow down the aging process, rescuing the brain as well as other organs from increased free radical damage, is to cut back on calories.

10. Take good care of yourself.

A more gentle approach to life can reduce chronic mental stress, which floods your brain inappropriately with adrenaline and other stress-activated chemicals that can actually inflict damage on neurons. Physical exercise, new research proves, improves blood flow to the brain and even perks up mental activity in specific parts of the brain. Keeping your blood vessels free of clogging and damage is essential to preserving brain function. That means controlling blood pressure, bad-type cholesterol, and the blood toxin homocysteine, all of which promote strokes and Alzheimer's disease. Stimulate your brain by learning and doing new things; such mental gymnastics actually encourage growth of new brain cell connections, enlarging memory and learning capacity.

The most important thing to remember is that your brain is growing and changing every instant. It thrives on stimulation, exercise, education, and the right diet and supplements. It is never too early or too late to decide to shape your own brain's destiny.

SELECTED REFERENCES

In writing *Your Miracle Brain*, I did extensive computer searches of the medical literature on Medline and of articles in major newspapers, magazines, and newsletters on Lexis-Nexis. I attended many scientific conference and/or read the proceedings and abstracts of such meetings, and interviewed numerous scientists in person, by phone, and e-mail. I also read many books on the functioning of the brain. Throughout the book I note sources for much of the information. For those who would like more precise scientific references, here are selected scientific journal articles out of the many that make up the sources for this book. They are listed alphabetically by first author.

Al Abed, Y., et al. Inhibition of advanced glycation end-product formation by actaldehyde: role in the cardio-protective effect of ethanol. *Proc Natl Acad Sci USA*; 96(5):2385–90, 1999.

Alpert, J.E., et al. Nutrition and depression: the role of folate. *Nutrition Reviews*; 55(5):145–149, 1997.

Amendola, C.A., et al. Caffeine's effects on performance and mood are independent of age and gender. *Nutritional Neuroscience*; 1(4):269–280, 1998.

Annadora J., et al. Food restriction reduces brain damage and improves behavioral outcome following excitotoxic and metabolic insults. *Ann Neurol*; 45:8–15, 1999.

Bell, I.R., et al. Relationship of normal serum vitamin B12 and folate levels to cognitive test performance in subtypes of geriatric major depression. *J Geriatr Psychiatry Neurol*; 3(2): 98–105, 1990.

Bendich, Adrianne, et al. Rationale for the introduction of long chain polyunsaturated fatty acids and for concomitant increase in the level of vitamin E in infant formulas. *International Journal of Vitamin and Nutrition Research*; 67:213–231, 1997.

Benton, David, and Haller, Jurg. The impact of long-term vitamin supplementation on cognitive functioning. *Psychopharmacology*; 117:298–305, 1995.

Benton, David, et al. Vitamin and mineral supplements improve the intelligence scores and concentration of six-year-old children. *Person Individ Diff*; 12(11):1151–1158, 1991.

Benton, David, et al. Selenium supplementation improves mood in a double-blind trial. *Psychopharmacology*; 102:549–550, 1990.

Benton, David, et al. The impact of long term vitamin supplementation on cognitive functioning. *Psychopharmacology*; 117:298–305, 1995

Benton, David, et al. Vitamin/mineral supplementation and intelligence. *Lancet*; 335 (8698)1158–1160, May 12, 1990.

Benton, David. Symposium on 'Nutrition and cognitive efficiency.' *Proceedings of the Nutrition Society*; 51:295–302, 1992.

Benton, David, et al. Vitamin and mineral supplements improve the intelligence scores and concentration of six-year-old children. *Person Individ Diff*; 12 (11):1151–1158, 1991.

Benton, David, et al. Effect of vitamin and mineral supplementation on intelligence of a sample of schoolchildren. *Lancet*;1 (8578): 140-143, 1988.

Benton, David, et al. Breakfast, blood glucose and cognition. *Am J Clin Nutr*; 67 (suppl):772S–778S, 1998.

Berger K., et al. Light-to-moderate alcohol consumptin and the risk of stroke among U.S. male physicians. *New England Journal of Medicine*; 34 (21): 1557–15 64, 1999.

Berr, Claudine, et al. Systemic oxidative stress and cognitive performance in the population-based Eva study. *Free Radical Biology & Medicine*; 24(7/8):1202–1208, 1998.

Bertelli A., et al. Carnitine and coenzyme Q10: biochemical proerties and functions, synergism and complementary action. *Int J Tiss Reac;* XII (3):183–186, 1990.

Birch, E.E., et al. Visual acuity and the essentiality of docosahexaenoic acid and arachidonic acid in the diet of term infants. *Pediatric Research*; 44(2):201–209, 1998.

Blaylock, Russell L. Neurogeneration and aging of the central nervous system: Prevention and treatment by phytochemicals and metabolic nutrients. *Integrative Medicine*;1(3):117–133, summer, 1998.

Blusztajn, J.K. Choline, a vital amine. *Science*; 281:794–795, August 7, 1998.

Bottiglieri, T. The clinical potential of ademetionine (S-adenosylmethionine) in neurological disorders. *Drugs*; 48(2):137–52, 1994.

Brattstrom, Lars. et al. Hyperhomocysteinemia in stroke: prevalence, cause and relationships to type of stroke and stroke risk factors. *Eur J Clin Invest* 22:214–221, 1992.

Brattstrom, Lars et al. Hyperhomocysteinemia as a risk factor for stroke. *Neurol Res*; 14(2 Suppl):81–84, 1992.

Brighenti, F. et al. Effect of neutralised vinegar and native vinegar on blood glucose and acetate responses in healthy subjects. *European Journal of Clinical Nutrition*; 49:242, 1995.

Brouwer, I.A. Low dose folic acid supplementation decreases plasma homocysteine concentrations: a randomized trial. *Am J Clin Nutr* 69:99–104, 1999.

Brighenti, F. et al. Effect of neutralised vinegar and native vinegar on blood glucose and acetate responses in healthy subjects. *European Journal of Clinical Nutrition*; 49:242, 1995.

Broadhurst, C.L., and Crawford, M.A. Rifts Valley lake fish and shellfish provided brain-specific nutrition for early Homo. *Br J Nutr*; 79(1):3–21, 1998

Cao, G., et al. Increases in human plasma antioxidant capacity after consumption of controlled diets high in frutis and vegetables. *American Journal of Clinical Nutrition*; 68:1081–67, 1998.

Carlson, Linda E., et al. Steroid hormones, memory and mood in a healthy elderly population . *Psychoneuroendocrinology*; 23(6):583–603, 1998.

Cenacchi, B., et al. Cognitive decline in the elderly: a double blind, placebo-controlled multicenter study on efficacy of phosphatidylserine administration. *Aging Clin Exp Res*; 5:123–133, 1993.

Chen, C., et al. Different effects of the constituents of EGb761 on apoptosis in rat cerebrellar granule cells induced by hydroxyl radicals. *Biochem Mol Biol Int*; 47(3):397–405, 1999.

Chomé, J., et al. Effects of suboptimal vitamin status on behavior,. *Biblthca Nutr Dieta*; 38:94–103, 1986.

Clarke, Robert. Lowering blood homocysteine with folic acid based supplements: meta-analysis of randomised trials. *British Medical Journal*; 316(7135):894, 1998.

Clarke, Robert, et al. Folate, vitamin B_{12} and serum total homocysteine levels in confirmed Alzheimer disease. *Arch Neurol* 55:1449–1455, 1998.

Connor, William E. Increased docosahexaenoic acid levels in human newborn infants by administration of sardines and fish oil during pregnancy. *Lipids*; 31 supplement: S–183–187, 1996.

Crook, T.H., et al. Effects of phosphatidylserine in age-associated memory impairment. *Neurology*; 41(5):644–649, 1991.

Dager, S.R., et al. Human brain metabolic response to caffeine and the effects of tolerance. *American Journal of Psychiatry*; 156:229–37, 1999.

Dai, J., et al. Recovery of axonal transport in "dead" neurons. *Lancet*; 351(9101):499–500, 1998.

Daviglus, M.L, et al. Dietary vitamin C, beta carotene and 30-year risk of stroke: results from the Western Electric Study. *Neuroepidemiology*; 16(2):69–77, 1997.

Davis, D.G., et al. Alzheimer neuropathologic alterations in aged cognitively normal subjects. *J Neuropathol Exp Neurol*; 58(4):376–88, 1999.

De Carli, C., et al. Predictors of brain morphology for the men of the NHLBI twin study. *Stroke*; 30:529–536, 1999.

de Rijk, M.C., et al. Dietary antioxidants and Parkinson's disease. The Rotterdam Study. *Arch Neurol* 54(6):762–5, 1997.

Deijen, J.B., et al. Vitamin B–6 supplementation in elderly men: effects on mood, memory, performance and mental effort. *Psychopharmacology*; 109:489–496, 1992.

di Tomaso, E., et al. Brain cannabinoids in chocolate. *Nature*; 382(6593):677–678, Aug. 22, 1996

Durlach, P.J. The effects of a low dose of caffeine on cognitive performance. *Psychopharmacology (Berl)*; 140(1):116–9, 1998.

Eaton, S.B. et al. An evolutionary perspective enhances understanding of human nutritional requirements. *Journal of Nutrition*, 126:1732–1740, 1996.

Edwards, Rhian, et al. Omega–3 polyunsaturated fatty acid levels in the diet and in red blood cell membranes of depressed patients. *J Affective Disorders*; 48:149–155, 1998.

Ernst, M., Zametkin, A.J., et al. Age related changes in brain glucose metabolism in adults with attention-deficit/hyperactivity disorder and control subjects. *J Neuropsychiatry Clin Neurosci Spring*; 10(2):168–77, 1998.

Evans, S.M. and Griffiths, R.R. Caffeine withdrawal: a parametric analysis of caffeine dosing conditions. *J Pharmacol Exp Ther*; 289(1):285–94, 1999.

Field, Barbara H. et al. Ginkgo biloba and memory: An overview. *Nutritional Neuroscience*; 1 255–267, 1998.

Finley, J.W. and Penland, J.G. Adequacy or deprivation of dietary selenium in healthy men: clinical and psychological findings. *Journal of Trace Elements in Experimental Medicine*; 11(1):17, 1998.

Fioravanti, M. et al. Low folate levels in the cognitive decline of elderly patients and the efficacy of folate as a treatment for improving memory deficits. *Archives of Gerontology and Geriatrics*; 26:1–13, 1997.

Gale, Catharine R. et al. Cognitive impairment and mortality in a cohort of elderly people. *British Medical Journal*; 312:608–11, 1996.

Gale, Catharine R. et al. Vitamin C and risk of death from stroke and coronary heart disease in a cohort of elderly people. *BMJ*; 310:1563–6, 1995.

Gillman, Matthew W. et al. Protective effect of fruits and vegeables on development of stroke in men. *JAMA*; 273(14):1113–1117, 1995.

Glueck C.J. et al. Improvement in symptoms of depression and in an index of life stressors accompany treatment of severe hypertriglyceridemia. *Biol Psychiatry*; 34(4):240–52, 1993.

Goodwin, James S. et al. Association between nutritional status and cognitive functioning in a healthy elderly population. *JAMA*; 249(21):2917–2921, 1983.

Gowri K., et al. Prenatal dietary choline supplementation decreases the threshold for induction of long-term potentiation in young adult rats. *J Neurophysiol*; 79:1790–1796, 1998.

Greenwood, C.E. et al. Cognitive impairment in rats fed high fat diets: A specific effect of saturated fatty acid intake. *Behav Neurosci*; 110:451–459, 1996.

Griffiths, R.R. Low dose caffeine discrimination in humans. *Journal of Pharmacology and Experimental Therapeutics*; 252(3):970–978, 1990.

Haan, Mary N. et al. The role of APOE e4 in modulating effects of other risk factors for cognitive decline in elderly persons. *JAMA*; 282(1):40–46, 1999.

Hachinski, V. et al. Lipids and stroke: a paradox resolved. *Arch Neurol Apr*; 53(4):303–8, 1996

Hagan T.M. et al. R-alipoic acid-supplemented old rats have improved mitochondrial function, decreased oxidative damage, and increased metabolic rate. *FASEB Journal*; 13:411–418, 1999.

Haller, J. Mental Health: Minimental State Examination and geriatric depression score of elderly Europeans in the SENECA study of 1993. *Eur J Clin Nutr*; 50 Suppl 2:S112–116, 1996.

Heiss, W.D. et al. Activation of PET as an instrument to determine therapeutic efficacy in Alzheimer's disease. *Annals NY Acad Sci*; 695:327–31, 1993.

Hamazaki, T. et al. The effect of docosahexaenoic acid on aggression in young adults. *Journal of Clinical Investigation*; 97:(4):1129–33, 1996: (4):1129–33, 1996.

Healton, E.B, et al. Neurologic aspects of cobalamin deficiency; Medicine (Baltimore): 70(4):229–45, 1991.

Heseker, H. et al. Psychological disorders as early symptoms of a mild-to-moderate vitamin deficiency. *Annals New York Academy of Sciences*; 669:352–357, 1992.

Hibbeln, J.R. Fish consumption and major depression. *Lancet*; 351:1213, 1998.

Hibbeln, J.R. et al. Dietary polyunsaturated fatty acids and depression: When cholesterol does not satisfy. *American Journal of Clinical Nutrition*; 62:1–9, 1995.

Hindmarch, I. et al. The effects of black tea and other beverages on aspects of cognition and psychomotor performance. *Psychopharmacology*; 139:230–238, 1999.

Hoffer, Abram. Gaining control of schizophrenia. *American Journal of Natural Medicine*; 5(5):21–25, 1998.

Horwood, L.J., et al. Breastfeeding and later cognitive and academic outcomes. *Pediatrics*; 101(1): E9, 1998.

Horrocks, Lloyd A., et al. Health benefits of docosahexaenoic acid (DHA.) *Pharmacol Res*; 40(3): 211–25, 1999.

Howard, Barbara V. Dietary fatty acids, insulin resistance, and diabetes. *Annals New York Academy of Sciences*; 215–220, 1997.

Hu, Frank B. et al. A prospective study of egg consumption and risk of cardiovascular disease in men and women. *JAMA*; 281(15):1387–1394, 1999.

Hyman, B.T. Neuronal loss in Alzheimer's disease. *Aging Clin Exp Res*; 10(2):156, 1998.

Jama, J. Warsama, et al. Dietary antioxidants and cognitive function in a population-based sample of older persons. The Rotterdam Study. *American Journal of Epidemiology*; 144:275–80, 1996.

James, Jack E. Acute and chronic effects of caffeine on performance, mood, headache and sleep. *Neuropsychobiology*; 38:32–41, 1998.

Johnson, D.L. et al. Breast feeding and children's intelligence. *Psychol Rep*; 79(3 Pt 2):1179–85, 1996.

Joseph, J.A. et al. Oxidative stress and age-related neuronal deficits. *Molecular and Chemical Neuropathology*; 28:35–40, 1996.

Joseph, J.A. et al. Long-term dietary strawberry, spinach, or vitamin E supplementation retards the onset of age-related neuronal signal transduction and cognitive behavioral deficits. *The Journal of Neuroscience*; 18(19): 8047–8055, 1998.

Joseph, J.A., et al. Reversals of age-related declines in neuronal signal transduction, cognitive and motor behavioral deficits with blueberry, spinach or strawberry dietary supplementation. *Journal of Neuroscience;* 19 (18): 8114–8121, September 15, 1999.

Kalmijn, S. et al. Polyunsaturated fatty acids, antioxidants, and cognitive function in very old men. *American Journal of Epidemiology*; 145:33–41, 1997.

Kaplan, Randall J., and Greenwood, Carold E. Dietary saturated fatty acids and brain function. *Neurochemical Research*; 23(5):615–626, 1998.

Keli, S.Q. et al. Dietary flavonoids, antioxidant vitamins and incidence of stroke: the Zutphen Study. *Arch Intern Med*; 156(6):637–42, 1996.

Kempermann, G. and Gage, Fred H. Closer to neurogenesis in adult humans. *Nature Medicine*; 4(5):555–557, 1998.

Khaw, K. Dietary potassium and stroke associated mortality. *New England Journal of Medicine*; 216:235–40, 1987.

Kilander, Lena et al. Hypertension is related to cognitive impairment. *Hypertension*; 31:780–786, 1998.

Kolb, Bryan, et al. Brain plasticity and behavior. *Annual Review of Psychology*; 49: 43, January 1, 1998.

Korol, D.L. and Gold, P.E. Glucose, memory and aging. *Am J Clin Nutr*; 67(suppl):764S–771S, 1998.

Kritchevsky, S.B. et al. Dietary antioxidants and carotid artery wall thickness: the ARIC study. *Circulation*; 92: 2142–2150, 1995.

Kubala, Albert L. et al. Nutritional factors in psychological test behavior (citrus fruit). *The Journal of Genetic Psychology*; 96:343–352, 1960.

La Rue, Asenath, et al. Nutritional status and cognitive functioning in a normally aging sample: a 6-year reassessment. *Am J Clin Nutr*; 65:20–9, 1997.

Lanting, C.I., et al. Neurological difference between 9-year-old children fed breast milk or formula-milk as babies. *Lancet*; 334:1319–22, 1994.

Launer, Lenore J., et al. The association between midlife blood pressure levels and late-life cognitive function. The Honolulu-Asia Aging Study. *JAMA*; 274: 1846–1851, 1995.

Le Bars, Pierre L. et al. A placebo controlled, double blind randomized trial of an extract of ginkgo biloba for dementia. *JAMA*; 278(16):1327–1332, 1997.

Lehto S. et al. Predictors of stroke in middle aged patients with non-insulin dependent diabetes. *Stroke*; 27(1):63–68, 1996.

Levi, B., et al. Long-term fructose consumption acclerates glycation and several age-related variables in male rats. *J Nutr*; 128(9):1442–9, 1998.

Lieberman, H.R., Wurtman, R.J., et al. The effects of low doses of caffeine on human performance and mood. *Psychopharmacology*; 92:308–312, 1987.

Ligeberg, H.G.M. et al. Delayed gastric emptying rate as a potential mechanism for lowered glycemia after eating sourdough bread. *Am J Clin Nutr*; 64:886, 1996.

Linko, Y.Y. et al. Docosahexaenoic acid: a valuable nutraceutical? *Trends in Food Science & Technology*; 7:59–63, 1996.

Logroscino, Giancarlo et al. Dietary lipids and antioxidants in Parkinson's disease: a population-based case-control study. *Ann Neurol*; 39:89–94, 1996.

Lonsdale, Derrick. Red cell transketolase studies in a private practice specializing in nutritional correction. *Journal of the American College of Nutrition*; 7(1):61–67, 1988.

Lonsdale, Derrick et al. Red cell transketolase as an indicator of nutritional deficiency. *Am J Clin Nutr*; 33:305–211, 1980.

Lucas, A. et al. Breast milk and subsequent intelligence quotient in children born preterm. *Lancet*; 339(8788): 261–264, 1992.

Lovell, M.A. et al. Elevated thiobarbituric acid-reactive substances and antioxidant enzyme activity in the brain in Alzheimer's disease. *Neurology*; 45(8):1594–1601, 1995.

Manson, J.E., et al. Vegetable and fruit consumption and incidence of stroke in women. *Circulation*; 89:932, 1994 (abstract).

Matthews, R.T. et al. Coenzyme Q10 administration increases brain mitochondrial concentrations and exerts neuroprotect effects. *Proceedings of the National Academy of Sciences*; 95(15):8892, 1998.

McDonald, R.B. Influence of dietary sucrose on biological aging. *Am J Clin Nutr*; 62(suppl):284S–293S, 1995.

Meck, Warren H. et al. Characterization of the facilitative effects of perinatal choline supplementation on timing and temporal memory. *NeuroReport*; 8:2831–2835, 1997.

Minami, M. et al. Dietary docosahexaenoic acid increases cerebral acetylcholine levels and improves passive avoidance performance in stroke-prone spontaneously hypertensive rats. *Pharmacol Biochem Behav*; 58: 1123–1129: 1997.

Morris, M.C. et al. Vitamin E and vitamin C supplement use and risk of incident Alzheimer Disease. *Alzheimer Dis Assoc Disord*; 12(3):121–126, 1998.

Mueller, E.A. et al. Brain volume preserved in healthy elderly through the eleventh decade. *Neurology*; 51:1555–1562, 1998.

Munch, G., et al. Advanced glycation endproducts in aging and Alzheimer's disease. *Brain Res. Brain Res Rev*; 23:134–143, 1997.

Murphy, J. Michael et al. The relationship of school breakfast to psychosocial and academic functioning. *Arch Pediatr Adolesc Med*; 152:899–907, 1998.

Neeper S.A. et al. Physical activity increases mRNA for brain derived neurotrophic factor and nerve growth factor in rat brain. *Brain Research*; 726(1–2):49–56, 1996.

Okuyama, Harumi, et al. Dietary fatty acids—the n–6/n–3 balance and chronic elderly diseases. Excess linoleic acid and relative n–3 deficiency syndrome seen in Japan. *Prog Lipid Res*; 35:409–457, 1997.

Orencia, A.J. et al. Fish consumption and stroke in men. 30-year findings of the Chicago Western Electric Study. *Stroke*; 27:204–209, 1996.

Ortega, R.M., et al. Dietary intake and cognitive function in a group of elderly people. *American Journal of Clinical Nutrition*; 66:803–809, 1997.

Packer, L. , et al. Antioxidant acivity and biologic properties of a procyanidin-rich extract from pine (Pinus Maritima) bark, pycnogenol. *Free Radical Biology and Medicine*; 32:704–724, 1999.

Packer, L. et al. Alpha lipoic acid—the metabolic antioxidant. *Free Radical Biology & Medicine*; 20:625–26, 1996.

Packer, L. et al. Neuroprotection by the metabolic antioxidant a-lipoic acid. *Free Radical Biology & Medicine*; 22(1–2):359–78, 1997.

Paleologos, Michael, et al. Cohort study of vitamin C intake and cognitive impairment. *Am J Epidemiol*; 148:45–50, 1998.

Peet, Malcolm. Depletion of omega–3 fatty acid levels in red blood cell membranes of depressive patients. *Biol Psychiatry*; 43:315–319, 1998.

Perkins, Anthony J. Association of antioxidants with memory in a multiethnic elderly sample using the Third National Health and Nutrition Examination Survey. *Am J Epidemiol*; 150:37–44, 1999.

Perrig, Walter J. et al. The relation between antioxidants and memory performance in the old and very old. *J Am Geriatr Soc*; 45:718–724, 1997.

Perry, I.J., et al. Prospective study of serum total homocysteine concentration and risk of stroke in middle aged British men. *Lancet*; 346:1395–98, 1995.

Pirttila, T., et al. Effect of advanced brain atrophy and vitamin deficiency on cognitive functions in non-demented subjects. *Acta Neurol Scand*; 87: 161–66, 1993.

Prasad, K.N. et al. Prostaglandins as putative neurotoxins in Alzheimer's disease. *Proceedings of the Society of Experimental and Biological Medicine*; 219:120–125, 1998.

Prior, Ronald L. et al. Antioxidant capacity and polyphenolic components of teas: implications for altering in vivo antioxidant status. *Proceedings of the Society for Experimental Biology and Medicine*; 220(4):255–261, 1999.

Pyapali, Gowri K., et al. Prenatal dietary choline supplementation decreases the threshold for induction of long-term potentiation in young adult rats. ;; 79(4): 1790–1796, 1998.

Richardson, Alexandra J., et al. Abnormal cerebral phospholipid metabolism in dyslexia indicated by phosphorus–31 magnetic resonance spectroscopy. *NMR in Biomedicine*; 10:309–314, 1997.

Riedel, W. et al. Caffeine attenuates scopolamine-induced memory impairment in humans. *Psychopharmacology (Berl)*; 122(2):158–68, 1995.

Riggs, Karen M. et al. Relations of vitamin B–12, vitamin B–6, folate, and homocysteine to cognitive performance in the normative aging study. *Am J Clin Nutr*; 63:306–14, 1996.

Riso, P., et al. Does tomato consumption effectively increase the resistance of lymphocyte DNA to oxidative damage? *Am. J Clin Nutr*; 69:712–718, 1999.

Robinson, K. et al. Low circulating folate and vitamin B6 concentrations: risk factors for stroke, peripheral vascular disease, and coronary artery disease. European COMAC Group. Circulation; 97(5):437–43, 1998.

Sacco, R.L., et al. The protective effect of moderate alcohol consumption on ischemic stroke. JAMA 281 (1): 53–60, 1999.

Sano, Mary, et al. A controlled trial of selegiline, alpha-tocopherol or both as treatment for Alzheimer's disease. *New England Journal of Medicine*; 336:1216–1222, 1997.

Sapolsky, R.M. . Why stress if bad for your brain. *Science*; 273:5276:749–50, 1996; and FASEB abstracts, 1999.

Schmidt, R. et al. Plasma antioxidants and cognitive performance in middle-aged and older adults: results of the Austrian stroke prevention study. *J Am Geriatr Soc*; 46(11): 1407–10, 1998.

Schmidt, R. et al. Magnetic resonance imaging white matter hyperintensities in clinically normal elderly individuals. *Stroke*; 27:2043–2047, 1996.

Schoenthaler, Stephen J. et al. Controlled trial of vitamin-mineral supplementation on intelligence and brain function. *Person Individ Diff*; 12(4):343–350, 1991.

Schoenthaler, Stephen J. et al. Controlled trials of vitamin-mineral supplementation: effects on intelligence and performance. *Person Individ Diff*; 12(4): 351–362, 1991.

Selhub J. et al. Vitamin status and intake as primary determinants of homocysteinemia in the elderly. *JAMA*; 270: 2693–98, 1994.

Serafini, M., et al. In vivo antioxidant effect of green and black tea in man. *Eur J Clin Nutr*; 50:28–32, 1996.

Shaywitz, Sally E., et al. Effect of estrogen on brain activation patterns in postmenopausal women during working memory tasks. *JAMA*; 281(13):1197–1202, 1999

Skolnick, A. Brain researchers bullish on prospects for preserving mental functioning in the elderly. *JAMA*; 267(16): 2154, 1992.

Skoog, I. The relationship between blood pressure and dementia: a review. *Biomed & Pharmacother*; 51: 367–375, 1997.

Snowdon, David A., et al. Antioxidants and reduced functional capacity in the elderly; findings from the Nun Study. *J Gerontol A Biol Sci Med Sci*; 51(1):10–16, 1996.

Snowdon, David A., et al. Brain infarction and the clinical expression of Alzheimer disease: The Nun Study. *JAMA*; 277 (10): 813–817, 1997.

Sokol, Ronald J. Vitamin E and neurologic function in man. Free Radical Biology & Medicine 6:189–207, 1989.

Solfrizzi, V. et al. High monounsaturated fatty acids intake protects against age-related cognitive decline. *Neurology*; 52:1563–1568, 1999.

Stevens, L.J, et al. Essential fatty acid metabolism in boys with attention deficit hyperactivity disorder. *Am J Clin Nutr*; 62:761–768, 1995.

Stoll, A.L. Omega–3 fatty acids in bipolar disorder: a preliminary double-blind, placebo-controlled trial. *Arch Gen Psychiatry*; 56 (5): 407–412, 1999.

Stoll, S., et al. The potent free radical scavenger a-lipoic acid improves memory in aged mice. Putative relationship to NMDA receptor deficits. *Pharmacol Biochem Behav*; 46: 799–805, 1993.

Tomeo, A.C., et al. Antioxidant effects of tocotrienols in patients with hyperlipidemia and carotid stenosis. *Lipids*; 30(12):1179–83, 1995

Truelsen, T. Intake of beer, wine and spirits and risk of stroke: the Copenhagen city heart study. *Stroke*; 29 (12):2467-2472, 1998.

Tun, P.A., et al. Cognitive and affective disorders in elderly diabetics. *Clin Geriatr Med*; 6(4):731–46, 1990.

Vallardita, C., et al. Multicentre clinical trial of brain phosphatidylserine in elderly subjects with mental deterioration. *Clin Trials J*; 24:84–93, 1987.

Wainwright, P.E., et al. A saturated fat diet during development alters dendritic growth in mouse brain. *Nutritional Neuroscience*; 1: 49–58, 1998.

Warburton, D.M. Effects of caffeine on cognition and mood without caffeine abstinence. *Psychopharmacology*; 119:66–70, 1995.

Waterhouse, A.L. Antioxidants in chocolate. *Lancet*; 348 (9030): 834, 1996.

Willatts, P., et al. Effect of long chain polyunsaturated fatty acids in infant formula on problem solving at 10 months of age. *Lancet*; 352:688–91, 1998.

Wickelgren, Ingrid. Tracking insulin to the mind: *Science*; 280(5363):517, 1998.

Winther, K., et al. Effects of ginkgo biloba extract on cognitive function and blood pressure in elderly subjects. *Current Therapeutic Research*; 59(12):881–888, 1998.

Yao, H. Decreased plasma tryptophan associated with deep white matter lesions in elderly subjects. *J Neurol Neurosurg Psychiatry*; 66:100–103, 1999.

Yehuda, S., et al. Essential fatty acids preparation (SR–3) improves Alzheimer's patients' quality of life. *Int J Neurosci*; 87:141–149, 1996.

Yehuda, S. et al. Fatty acids and brain peptides. *Peptides*; 19(2):407–419, 1998

Yokota, A. relationship of polyunsatruated fatty acid composition and learning ability in rat. *Nippon Sanfujinka Gakkaishi*; 45:15–22, 1996.

Young, S.N. Folic acid and psychopathology. *Prog. Neuro-Psychopharmacol & Biol Psychiat*; 13:841–863, 1989.

Yudkin, John. Intelligence of children and vitamin-mineral supplements: the DRF study. Discussion, conclusion and consequences. *Personality and Individual Differences*; 12:363–5, 1991.

BOOKS

Ackerman, Sandra for the Institute of Medicine, National Academy of Sciences. *Discovering the Brain*. Washington, D.C., National Academy Press, 1992.

Benton, David. *Food for Thought*. London, Penguin Books, 1996.

Blaylock, Russell L. *Excitotoxins: The Taste that Kills*. Santa Fe, Health Press, 1997.

Brand-Miller, Jennie and Wolever, Thomas. *The Glucose Revolution*. New York, Marlowe & Company, 1999.

Brown, Richard; Bottiglieri, Teodoro; and Colman, Carol. *Stop Depression Now*. New York, G.P. Putnam's Sons, 1999.

Carper, Jean. *Stop Aging Now!* New York, HarperCollins, 1996.

Carper, Jean. *Food—Your Miracle Medicine*. New York, HarperCollins, 1993.

Carper, Jean. *Miracle Cures*. New York, HarperCollins, 1998.

Christensen, Larry. *Diet-Behavior Relationships*. Washington, D.C., American Psychological Association, 1996.

Conners, C. Keith. *Feeding the Brain*. New York, Plenum, 1989.

Crook, Thomas H. and Adderly, Brenda. *The Memory Cure*. New York, Pocket Books, 1998.

Diamond, Marian, Ph.D., and Hopson, Janet. *Magic Trees of the Mind: How to Nurture Your Child's Intelligence, Creativity and Healthy Emotions*. New York, Dutton, 1998.

Harman, Denham; Holliday, Robin; and Meydani, Mohsen, editors. *Towards Prolongation of the Healthy Life Span*. Annals of the New York Academy of Sciences, volume 854, New York, 1998.

Kotulak, Ronald. *Inside the Brain: Revolutionary Discoveries of How the Mind Works*. Kansas City, Andrews McMeel Publishing, 1996.

Lombard, Jay and Germano, Carl. *The Brain Wellness Plan*. New York, Kensington, 1997.

Masters, Roger D. and McGuire, Michael T. *The Neurotransmitter Revolution*. Carbondale, Ill., Southern Illinois University Press, 1994.

Packer, Lester. *The Antioxidant Miracle*. New York, John Wiley & Sons, Inc., 1999.

Packer, Lester; Hiramatsu, Midori; and Yoshikawa, Toshikazu. *Free Radicals in Brain Physiology and Disorders*. San Diego, Academic Press, 1996.

Papas, Andres. *The Vitamin E Revolution*. New York, HarperCollins, 1999.

Rosenthal, Norman. *St. John's Wort*. New York, HarperCollins, 1998.

Schmidt, Michael A. *Smart Fats*. Berkeley, California, Frog, Ltd., 1997.

Woodruff-Pak, Diana S. *The Neuropsychology of Aging*. Malden, Mass., Blackwell Publishers, Inc., 1997.

INDEX

dietary fat and insulin
resistance, 55–57
chocolate, 167–69
cholesterol. *See also* HDL
cholesterol
dietary fat and insulin
resistance and, 56
choline, 9, 202, 284–91
Christensen, Larry, 138–40, 189
chromium, 202
as an antioxidant, 133–34,
138–40
recommended levels of, 221
Clarke, Robert, 309
coenzyme Q10, 144, 147, 173,
260–67
ALS and, 264
antioxidant activity of,
260–61, 335–36
brain function and, 261–63
Parkinson's disease and,
265–66
recommended levels of, 266
coffee. *See* caffeine
Coffey, Edward, 18
Cognex, 234, 293
cognitive function. *See*
intellectual function
cola, 137, 180, 181, 187, 191
Coleman, Paul D., 23
computerized tomography (CT)
scans, 3
Connor, William E., 97–98
Cook, Richard, 200
corn oil, 50, 64, 65, 66, 73, 339
corticosteroids, 28
cortisol, and brain function, 28,
139
Cotman, Carl, 14, 35, 36, 232
Cott, Jerry, 84, 268, 271
Craft, Suzanne, 119
Crawford, Michael, 67–68

C-reactive protein (CRP), 332
Crook, Thomas H., III, 277–78,
279–80, 281, 282

dairy products, 41, 45
Davies, Peter, 19
DeCarli, Charles, 318–19
dementia
education level and, 32, 33, 34
folic acid and, 210, 213
glucose problems and, 108
insulin and, 120
meat consumption and,
171–72
memory and cognitive
changes in, 19
neurotransmitters and, 9–11
red wine and, 169
vascular, 305–6
dendrites, 5, 6, 11, 20
aging and, 12
dietary fat and, 48, 53
estrogen and growth of, 30
exercise and, 35
fish oil and, 69, 70
stimulation and growth of, 31,
32, 33–34
stress and, 28
depression, 207
caffeine and, 183–84
flaxseed oil and, 80–81
folic acid, 209, 210–11, 214,
308
glucose and chromium in,
138
homocysteine levels and, 308
omega-3 fat and, 68, 72, 78,
79, 81–82, 316
St. John's wort and, 295–98
SAM-e ("Sammy") and,
299–303
serotonin and, 10, 72

INDEX

manic depression, and fish oil,
81–82
Manning, Carol, 112
Manson, JoAnn E., 324
Markesbery, William R., 24
Mattson, Mark, 21, 172, 174, 175,
176, 232
Mayeux, Richard, 52, 175–76
Mazurek, Alan, 294
meats, 47
homocysteine levels and, 314
in Stone-Age diet, 41, 42, 44
memory
aging brain and, 14, 16–17,
19, 22
antioxidants and, 21, 22,
157–61, 162
blood sugar levels and,
109–11, 114–15, 118
brain stimulation and, 32
caffeine and, 181–82
choline and, 285–86, 288–89
dietary fat and, 50–51, 53,
62–63, 65
estrogen and, 29–30
fish oil and, 88
folic acid and, 211–12
glucose problems and, 108,
136
high blood pressure and,
317–18
homocysteine levels and, 308
huperzine and, 292–94
insulin resistance and, 53–54,
56
lipoic acid and, 255–56
neurotransmitters and, 8, 9
niacin and, 228–29
omega-3 fat and, 68
phosphatidylserine (PS) and,
278–80
selenium and, 252

serotonin and, 10
vitamin B$_6$ and, 215–17
vitamin deficiency and, 207
mental function, *see also*
intellectual function
fish oil and, 83–84
methylfolate, 209–10
Meyer, John Stirling, 35
mild cognitive impairment (MCI),
235–36, 271
milk and milk products, 41, 45
minerals, in Stone-Age diet, 46
mineral supplements, 47
brain function and, 334–35
intelligence levels and,
198–202
mitochondria
coenzyme Q10 and, 261, 262
DHA and, 74
free radicals in aging and,
19–20
glucose absorption and, 107–8
lipid peroxidation and, 144
lipoic acid and, 254
niacin and, 229
monounsaturated fat, 50, 131
mood
blood sugar and, 138–40
caffeine use and, 184
diet and, 7
glucose and, 108, 109
neurotransmitters and, 8
St. John's wort and, 296–97
selenium and, 250–52
serotonin and, 10
thiamin and, 223–24
triglycerides and, 312–15
vitamin B$_6$ and, 215
vitamin deficiency and, 207
multivitamins
brain function and, 203–5,
334–35

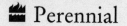 Perennial

Books by Jean Carper:

YOUR MIRACLE BRAIN
Maximize Your Brainpower • Boost Your Memory • Lift Your Mood
• Improve Your IQ and Creativity • Prevent and Reverse Mental Aging
ISBN 0-06-098440-6

Miraculous yet simple ways to maximize your brain power, improve your memory
and mood, and achieve peak mental, physical, and emotional performance by
utilizing the latest research in "nutritional neuroscience".

"[Your Miracle Brain] **turns complex, scientific research into exciting and
fascinating reading that will give hope and comfort to millions of people."**
—Norman Rosenthal, M.D., National Institute of Mental Health

STOP AGING NOW!
The Ultimate Plan for Staying Young and Reversing the Aging Process
ISBN 0-06-098500-3

Antioxidant vitamins, minerals, herbs and food chemicals are the magic youth
potion humans have been seeking for centuries. Carper reveals that much of what
we call aging can be prevented and reversed by supplements and foods.

"[Stop Aging Now!] **will add to the public's education about nutrition, disease,
and aging."**—Robert Butler, M.D., Mount Sinai School of Medicine

MIRACLE CURES
Dramatic New Scientific Discoveries Revealing the Healing
Powers of Herbs, Vitamins, and Other Natural Remedies
ISBN 0-06-098436-8

A breakthrough book that presents scientific evidence on the effectiveness
of natural remedies—culled from the world's leading doctors and scientists,
research centers, and major international scientific journals and combined with
awe-inspiring first-person medically verified accounts.

"Miracle Cures **will give herbal medicine a major boost in the minds of all
Americans."**—Mark Blumenthal, American Botanical Council

FOOD—YOUR MIRACLE MEDICINE
ISBN 0-06-098424-4

Caper shows how everybody can use food to prevent and cure more than 100
health problems from the common cold to cancer.

**"Provocative and filled with recent nutritional studies . . . there's a wealth of
useful information in this book."**—*USA Today*

Available wherever books are sold, or call 1-800-331-3761 to order.

Listen to

YOUR MIRACLE BRAIN

as read by the author

JEAN CARPER

". . . Carper is a pro behind the microphone. She reads with ease,
sounding much like a friendly relative offering advice."
— *Los Angeles Times*

ISBN 0-694-52189-2 • $18.00 ($26.95 Can.)
3 Hours • 2 Cassettes

And don't miss Carper's other audio books:

STOP AGING NOW!

ISBN 0-694-51581-7• $12.00 ($17.00 Can.)
1.5 Hours • 1 Cassette

MIRACLE CURES

ISBN 0-694-51848-4 • $12.00 ($17.00 Can.)
1.5 Hours • 1 Cassettes

Available wherever books are sold call 1-800-331-3761 to order.

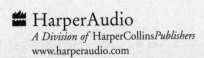
HarperAudio
A Division of HarperCollins*Publishers*
www.harperaudio.com